Breast Cancer Biology

Edited by Dil Afroze, Bilal Rah, Shazia Ali, Faheem Shehjar, Mohd Ishaq Dar, Shailender S. Chauhan and Natasha Thakur

Published in London, United Kingdom

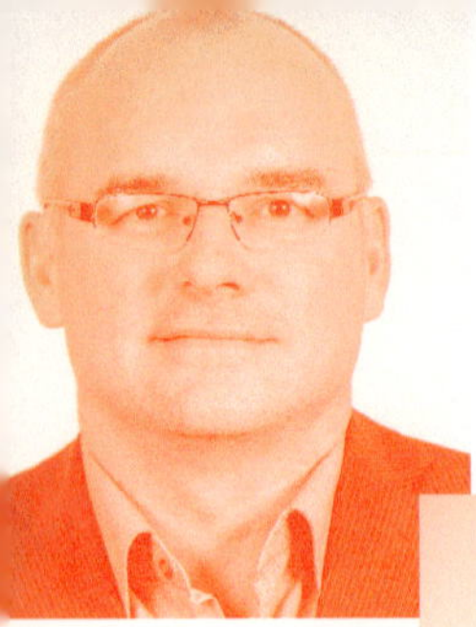
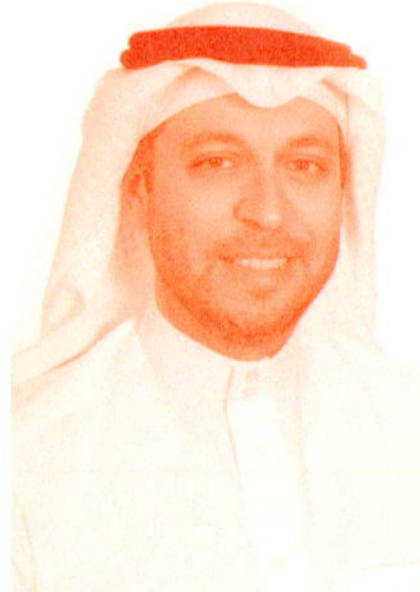
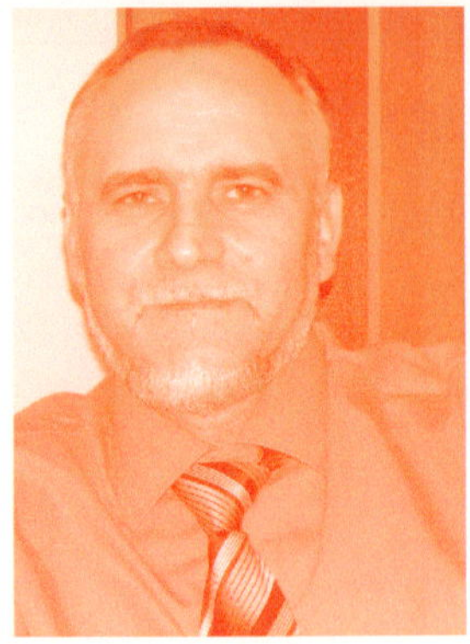
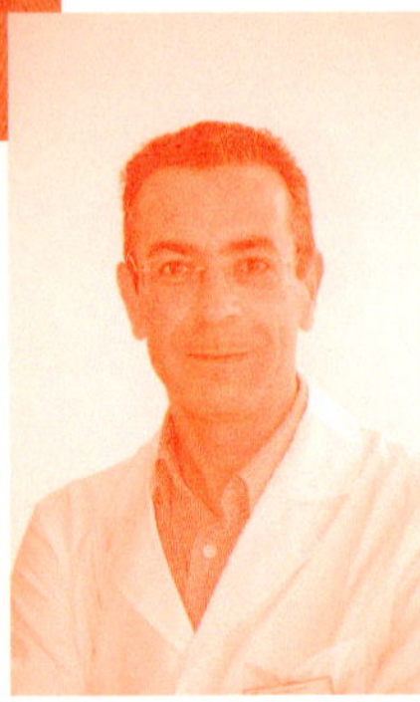
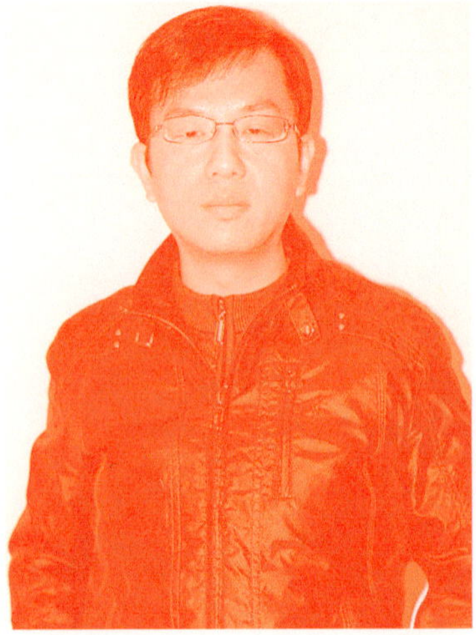
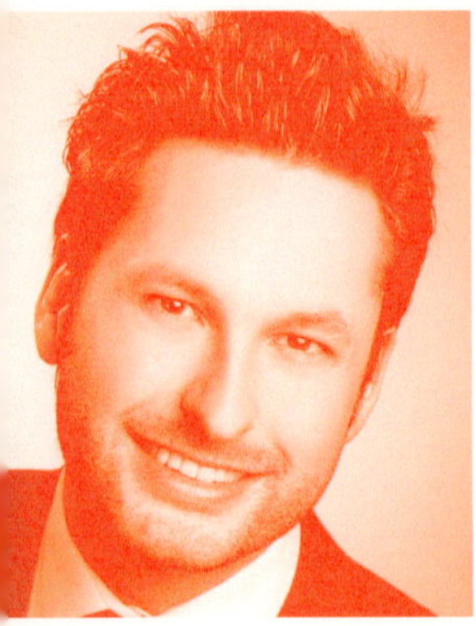
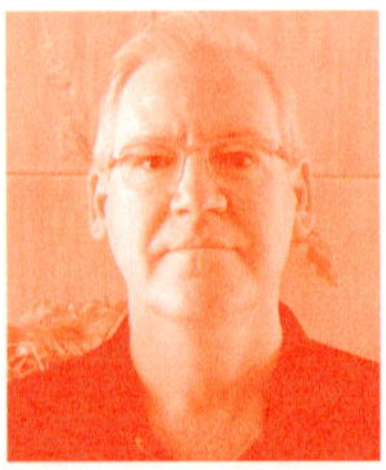

IntechOpen

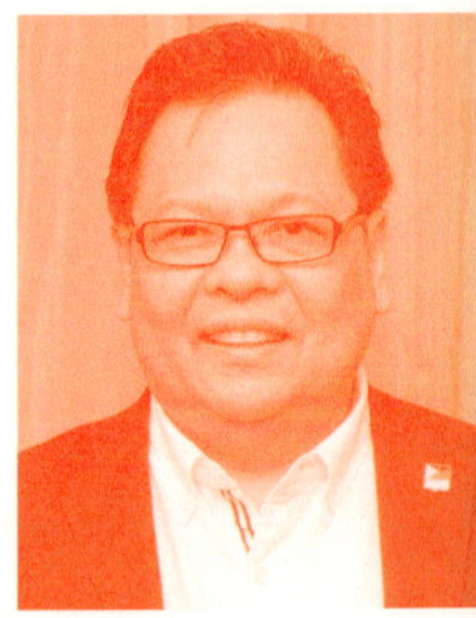
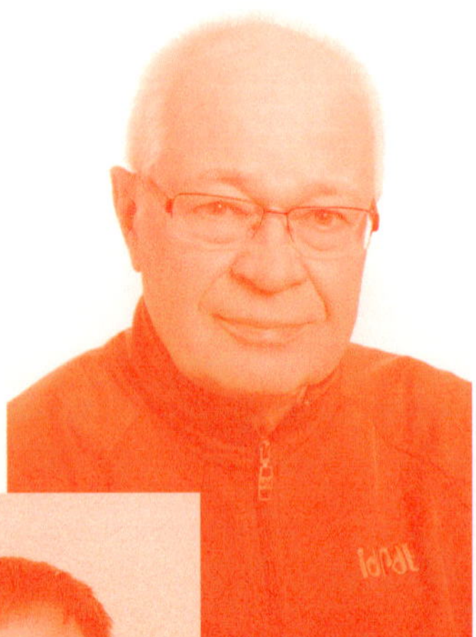
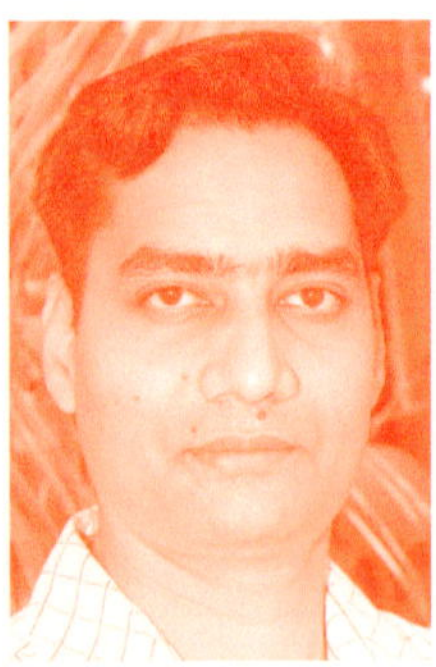
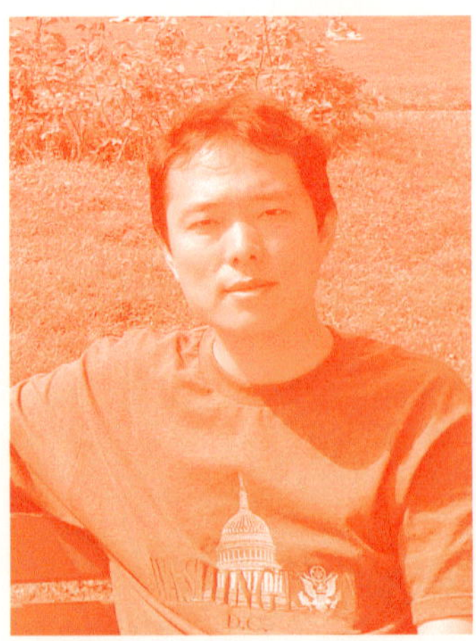
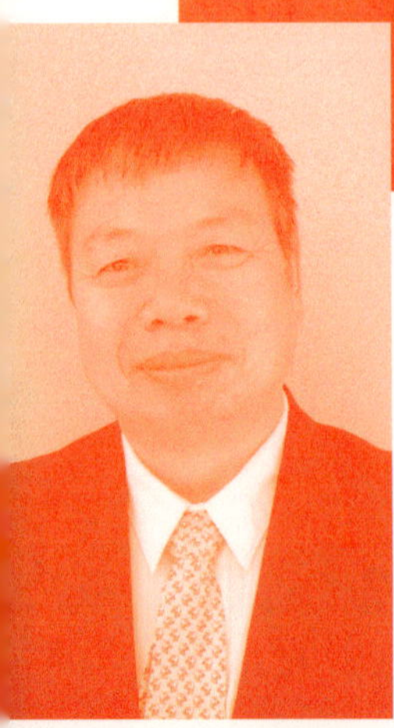
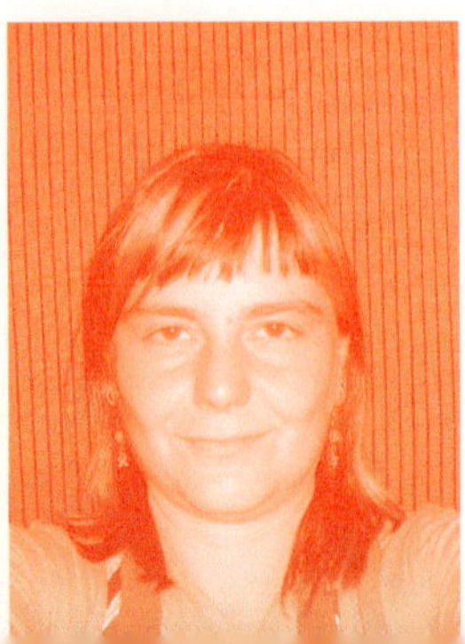

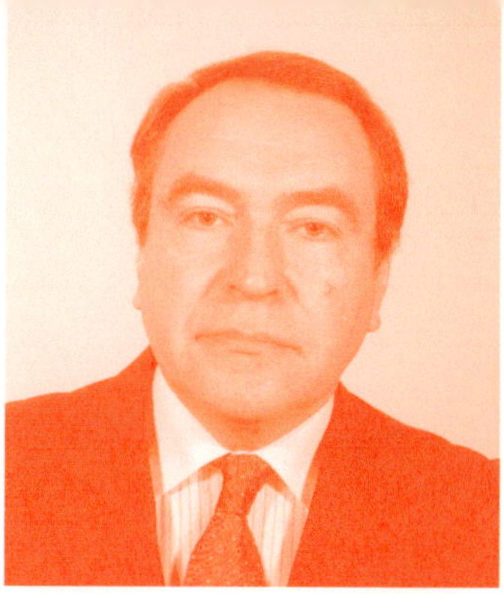
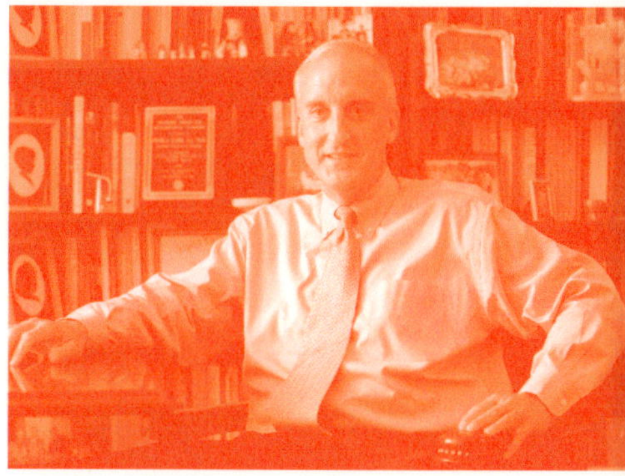
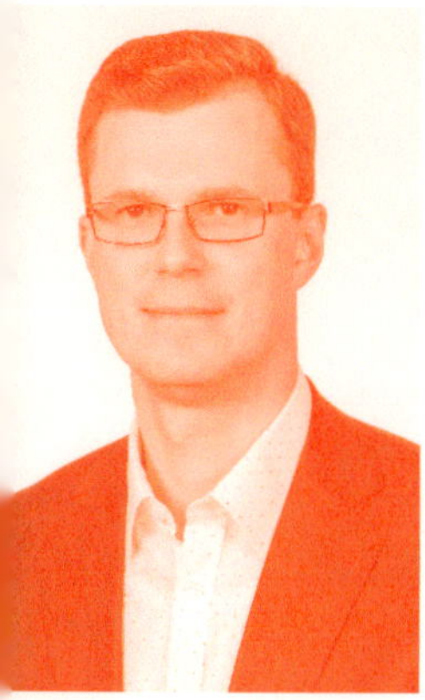
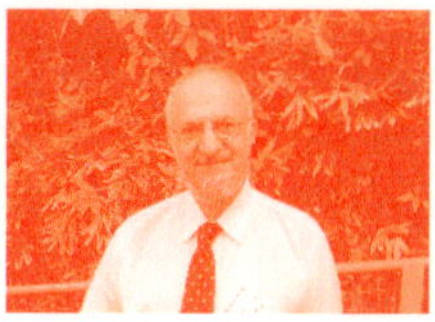
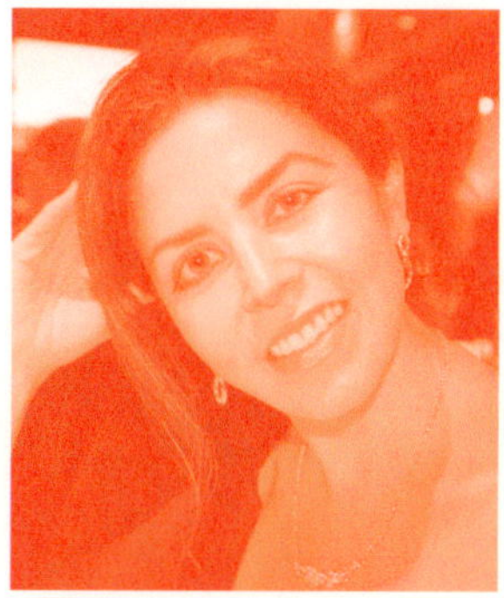

Supporting open minds since 2005

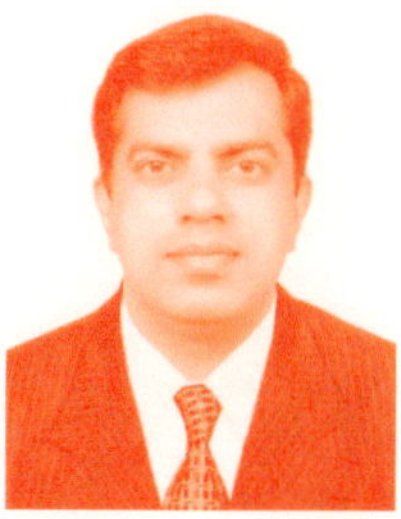
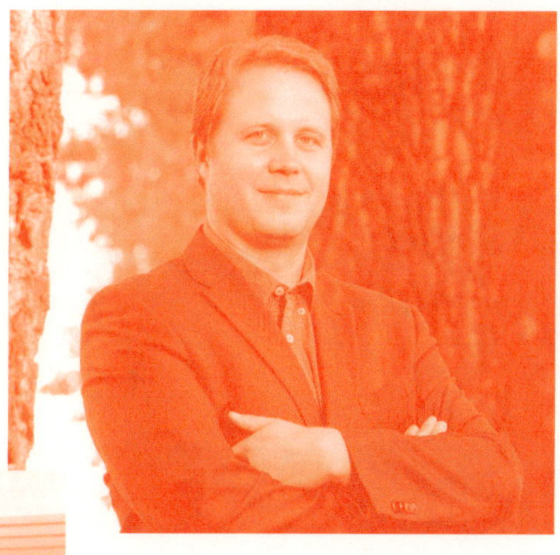
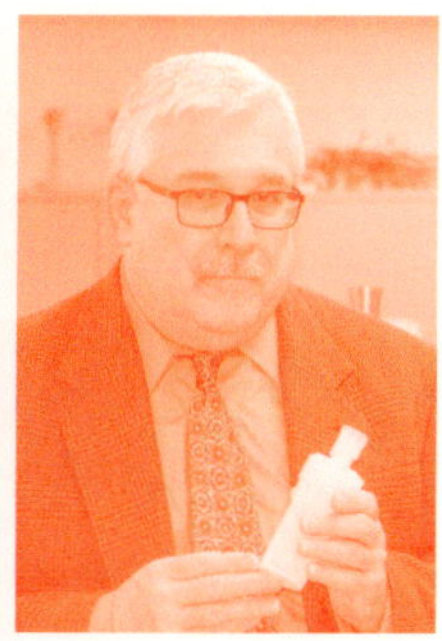
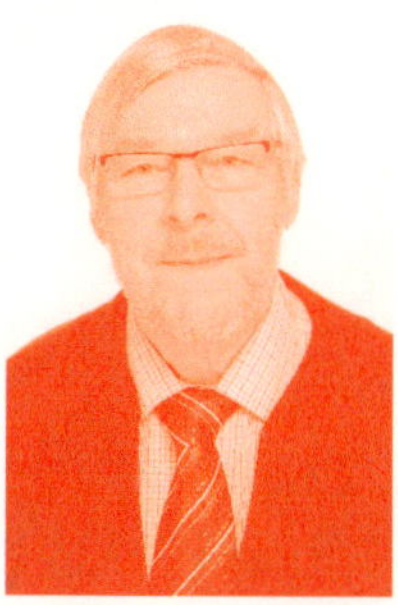
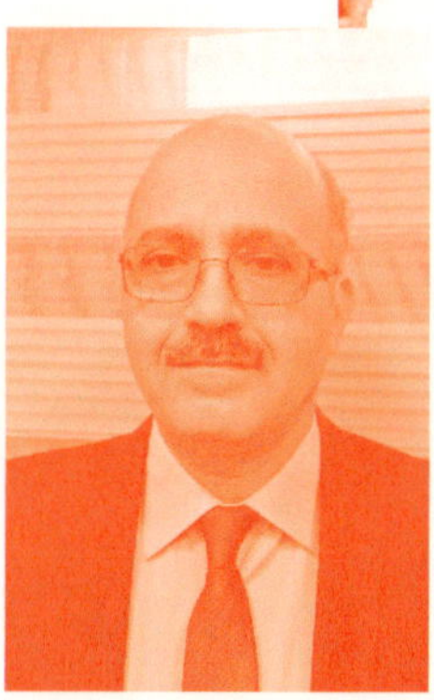
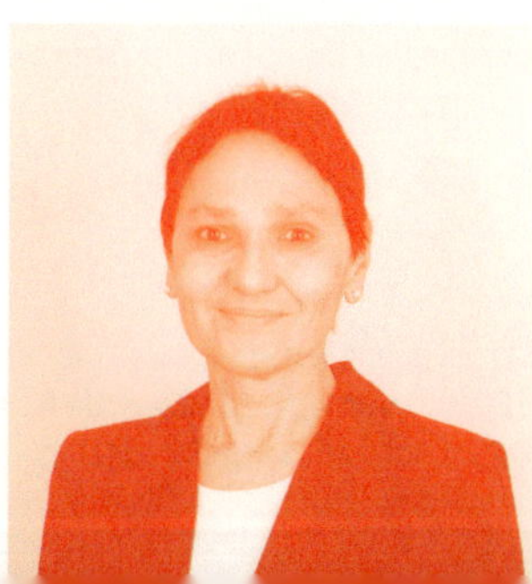
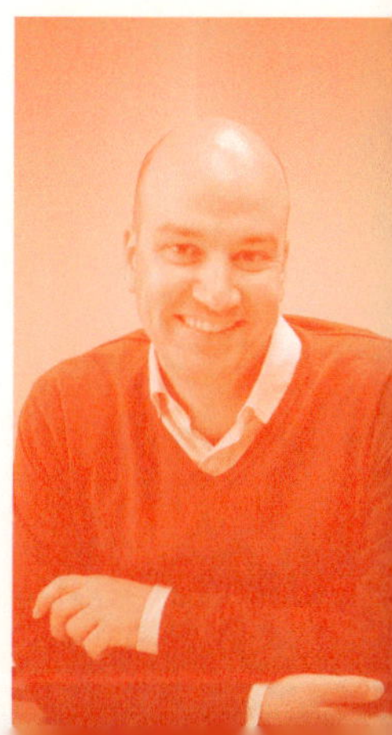

Breast Cancer Biology
http://dx.doi.org/10.5772/intechopen.78163
Edited by Dil Afroze, Bilal Rah, Shazia Ali, Faheem Shehjar, Mohd Ishaq Dar, Shailender S. Chauhan and Natasha Thakur

Contributors
Dingan Zhou, Deniz Kocamaz, Tülin Düger, Nagendra Ningaraj, Divya Khaitan, Ivan Mfouo-Tynga, Heidi Abrahamse, Veronique Maguer-Satta, Boris Guyot, Shazia Ali, Dil Afroze, Xing Zeng, Yadong Li, Zhixiong Wu, Xin Wan

First published in London, United Kingdom, 2020 by IntechOpen
IntechOpen is the global imprint of INTECHOPEN LIMITED, registered in England and Wales, registration number: 11086078, 7th floor, 10 Lower Thames Street, London, EC3R 6AF, United Kingdom
Printed in Croatia

British Library Cataloguing-in-Publication Data
A catalogue record for this book is available from the British Library

Additional hard and PDF copies can be obtained from orders@intechopen.com

Breast Cancer Biology
Edited by Dil Afroze, Bilal Rah, Shazia Ali, Faheem Shehjar, Mohd Ishaq Dar, Shailender S. Chauhan and Natasha Thakur
p. cm.
Print ISBN 978-1-78923-961-4
Online ISBN 978-1-78923-962-1
eBook (PDF) ISBN 978-1-78985-883-9

For EU product safety concerns:
IN TECH d.o.o., Prolaz Marije Krucifikse Kozulić 3, 51000 Rijeka, Croatia, info@intechopen.com or visit our website at intechopen.com.

Meet the editors

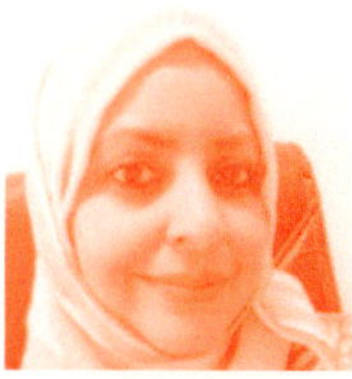

Dil Afroze (Ph.D) is a Professor and Chair at the Advanced Centre for Human Genetics, Sher-I-Kashmir Institute of Medical Sciences (SKIMS), India. After obtaining her doctorate from Jamia Millia Islamia, India, she joined the Department of Immunology and Molecular Medicine at SKIMS as faculty in 2005. With over two decades teaching experience in immunology and molecular medicine, Professor Dil Afroze is the Vice President of the Indian Immunology Society. She has been a registered guide for basic and clinical graduate and post graduate programs and has mentored postdoctoral fellows as well. She has a number of awards and honors to her credit at the national and international level. She has publications in high impact journals such as Frontiers, the International Journal of Infectious Disease, and the Journal of Chemical Biochemistry and is an editorial board member of several international books (IntechOpen publications). She has been a Visiting Professor in the Division of Oncology, University of Linköping, Sweden and Department of Anatomical Sciences and Neurobiology, University of Louisville School of Medicine, USA.

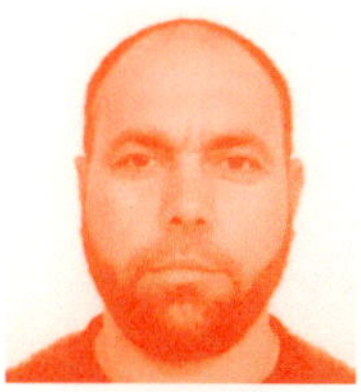

Dr. Bilal Ahmad Rah is an Assistant Professor (research) at Qasim University, Saudi Arabia. After obtaining his doctorate from the Academy of Scientific and Innovative Research (AcSIR)-IIIM, India, Dr. Rah's employment and positions include: Senior Resident, Sher-I-Kashmir Institute of Medical Sciences (SKIMS), Srinagar, India (2017); Post-Doctoral Research Associate, Comprehensive Cancer Centre, Ohio State, University, Columbus, Ohio, USA (2017); Post-Doctoral Research Associate, Buffet and Pamela Cancer Centre, University of Nebraska, Omaha, Nebraska, USA (2016); Best Paper award in Biology from the Indian Institute of Integrative Medicine, India (2015); Adhoc Assistant Professor, Department of Higher Education, India (2016). Dr. Rah is a member of the Indian Association of Cancer Research and an editorial board member of Journal Advances in Biomedicine and Pharmacy and co-editorship at IntechOpen Publications. His expertise includes cancer biology and genetics.

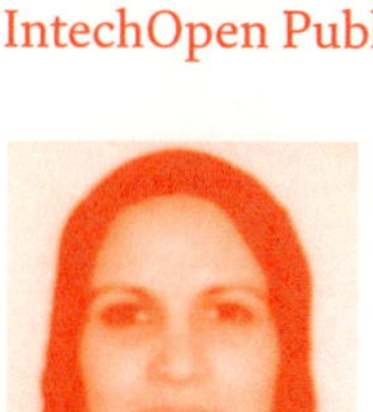

Dr. Shazia Ali is a Senior Resident at the Advanced Centre for Human Genetics, (SKIMS). After obtaining her doctorate from Life Sciences at Jawaharlal Nehru University, India, Dr. Ali's employment and positions include: Post-Doctoral Fellow DST, SKIMS (Nov 2016); Junior Residency, SKIMS (May 2016); Project Fellow, Indian Institute of Science, Bangalore India (2006-2008); Project Fellow, National Centre for Biological Sciences, Bangalore, India (2008); and Summer fellowship, Jawaharlal Nehru Centre for Advanced Research, Bangalore, India (2006). Dr. Ali is a member of the Indian Association of Cancer Research and a reviewer for Tumor Biology and a guest editor in the Sage Group of publications including co-editorship at IntechOpen Publications. Her expertise includes cancer biology, genetics and array hybridization.

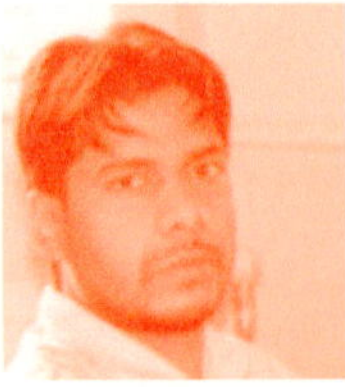

Dr. Faheem Shehjar is a Senior Resident at the Advanced Centre of Human Genetics (SKIMS). He obtained his doctorate in Biomedical Sciences from SKIMS (2017). He has also been a Senior Research Fellow at SKIMS (2017). Dr. Shehjar was awarded Exemplary Researcher Award, SKIMS (2018). Dr. Shehjar has published his research in various international reputed journals and has extensive experience in medical genetics and immunology and holds co-editorship at IntechOpen Publications. His expertise includes immunology and genetics.

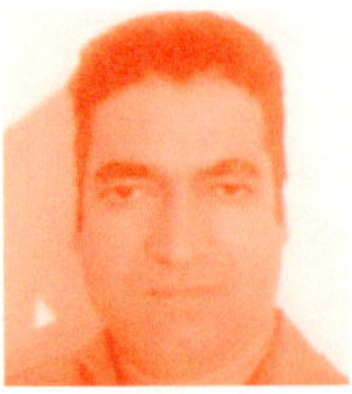

Dr. Mohd Ishaq Dar is a Senior Resident at the Advanced Centre of Human Genetics (SKIMS). He obtained his doctorate from the Academy of Scientific and Innovative Research (AcSIR)-IIIM, India. Dr. Ishaq's employment and positions include: Adhoc Assistant Professor at Department of Higher Education, India (2016). Dr. Mohd Ishaq Dar has published his research in various international reputed journals and holds several international patents. Dr. Ishaq is a member of the Indian Association of Cancer Research and is an editorial board member of the Journal Advances in Biomedicine and Pharmacy and holds co- editorship at IntechOpen Publications. His expertise includes cancer biology, stem cell biology, and epigenetics.

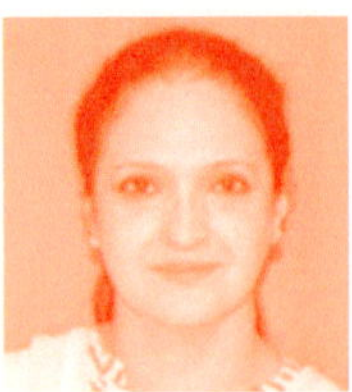

Dr. Natasha Thakur (M.D) is an Associate Professor at the Department of General Surgery, Sher-i-Kashmir Institute of Medical Sciences (SKIMS), India. She received her M.S at the Government Medical College, Jammu, J&K, India in 2004 and M.B.B.S at the University of Karnataka, India in 1994. Her previous positions and honors include: Surgeon Specialist DHS, Jammu, J&K,India (2005-08); Registrar Surgery, ASCHOMS, Batra Jammu, J&K, India (2004-05). Her previous employments include: Assistant Professor, General Surgery, SKIMS, Srinagar, J&K, India (2013-17) and Senior Resident, General Surgery, SKIMS, Srinagar, J&K, India (2008-13). Dr. Thakur has a Fellowship in gastrointestinal and endo surgery (FIAGES); Fellowship in breast cancer, AVON Global Scholar Program 2014, Atlanta, USA; and basic laparoscopic and advance suturing course. She is also a life member of the Association of Surgeons of India and Association of Colon and Rectal Surgeons of India.

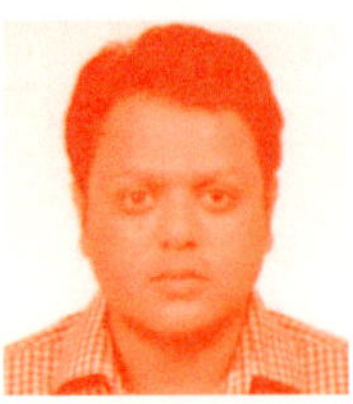

Dr. Shailender S. Chauhan is currently a Research Technician at the University of Arizona, Cancer Center, Tucson, AZ, USA. He received his PhD. in Biochemistry in 2013 from Panjab University, Chandigarh, India and M.Sc. (with Honors) in Biochemistry in 2005, also from Panjab University, Chandigarh, India. Dr. Chauhan has 9 publications, 2 manuscripts in the writing process, and 14 selected abstracts published in conference proceedings. He has received many national and international awards. Dr. Chauhan is an editorial board member and guest reviewer of various publications.

Contents

Preface

Breast Cancer Biology systematically describes breast cancer from basic definitions, to cellular and molecular biology, to diagnosis and treatment. This book also has some added focus on preclinical and clinical results in diagnosis and treatment of breast cancer. The book starts with an introduction on genetics, survival, and pathophysiology of breast cancer in Section 1. In Section 2, the molecular and cellular biology of breast cancer is presented with definite signaling pathways, especially the existence of breast cancer hypoxia. In Section 3, some new diagnostic methods and updated therapies from surgery, chemotherapy, hormone therapy, immunotherapy, radiotherapy, and some complementary therapies are discussed. Section 4 is focused on diet, exercise and other lifestyle factors for breast cancer prevention. This book provides a brief yet comprehensive overview of breast cancer for advanced students, graduate students, and researchers as well as those working with breast cancer in a clinical setting.

This book is a splendid compilation of six subjects associated with cancer covering a whole range of areas including breast cancer, signaling, genetics, mutation, cancer surviving, PI3K, AKT, Micro-RNA, chemo-resistance, hypoxia, and angiogenesis. Historically, prognosis and treatment choice making for breast cancer patients have been dictated by the anatomic amount of tumor spread. However, recently, breast cancer has become an assemblage of distinctive phenotypes with diverse prognoses, outlines of failure, and treatment responses. This book shows how biologically based assays and targeted therapies planned to exploit these unique phenotypes have intensely altered systemic therapy practice patterns and treatment consequences. This book aims to summarize the present data and provide practical framework for the integration of breast tumor biology into clinical practice.

Studies regarding ethnic, cultural, and personal differences in health beliefs and health care seeking behavior will yield important information for those providing care and setting policies. Also necessary is accurate, reliable, unbiased information on direct and indirect costs associated with genetic testing, prevention strategies, screening and diagnostic techniques, or a given treatment; such information is a critical component of realistic health care planning and delivery. An area of urgent importance is the effect of managed care on breast cancer screening, detection, treatment, and follow-up. There is concern about the trade-off between quality and cost of health care.

This book is covering a comprehensive range of topics. It has been a delightful opportunity to edit this special edition along with team of co-editors. We greatly appreciate the work of all the contributors to this book and they have brought with them a remarkable diversity of perspectives and fields that is truly reflective of the complexity of the topic, and they have come together in this project to create a node of multidisciplinary collaboration in this field.

We acknowledge the thousands of cancer patients who have participated in the studies, and who have inspired us to gather information leading to significant progress in knowledge in the field in the recent years.

We acknowledge the support of the Human Genetics Centre and associated Hospital, Sher-I-Kashmir Institute of Medical Sciences, Director, SKIMS, India.

Dr. Dil Afroze, Dr. Shazia Ali, Dr. Faheem Shehjar, Dr. Mohd Ishaq Dar and Dr. Natasha Thakur
Sher-I-Kashmir Institute of Medical Sciences,
India

Dr. Bilal Rah
Department of Medical Biotechnology,
College of Applied Medical Science,
Qassim University,
Kingdom of Saudi Arabia

Dr. Shailender S. Chauhan
University of Arizona,
USA

Section 1

Introduction on Breast Cancer Governed by Factors, Cell Cycle, Initiation and Progression

Chapter 1

Cell Cycle and Factors Involved in Inhibition or Progression of Breast Cancer

Shazia Ali, Mohd Ishaq Dar, Rafiq A. Rather and Dil Afroze

Abstract

Cell cycle progression is driven by the sequential activation of a family of cyclin-dependent kinases (CDKs), which phosphorylate and activate proteins that execute events critical to cell cycle progression. Cell cycle checkpoints are scrutiny points that display the order, integrity, and fidelity of the major proceedings of the cell cycle. These comprise development to the correct cell size, the replication, integrity of the chromosomes, and their precise separation at mitosis. Many of these mechanisms are prehistoric in origin and highly preserved and hence have been deeply well versed by studies in model organisms such as the yeasts as well as in higher organisms. These molecular mechanisms switch alternative cell fates with substantial impact on tumor suppression. In the present study, we have explained different checkpoint pathways and the consequences of their dysfunction on cell fate in cancer.

Keywords: cell cycle, breast cancer, drug resistance, tumor suppressor genes, oncogenes

1. Introduction

Deregulation in cell cycle is a remarkable feature of tumor cells [1, 2]. Cell cycle helps to maintain homeostasis of normal cell growth and viability in a compact process. Cell cycle occurs in four phases as follows:

- preparation for cell division in G1 phase;
- process of DNA synthesis in S phase;
- G2 phase for cell growth and enzyme production; and
- mitosis: M phase, which is regulated by several controlled events, directs the replication of DNA and cell division [3].

The transitions between G1 to S and G2 to M phase are governed by changes in the kinase activity of CDKs [4]: Cdk1, Cdk2, Cdk4, Cdk6, and cyclins. Cyclins are the regulatory units, and CDKs contain the catalytic subunit of an activated heterodimer. The cyclin binds to CDKs and gets activated by forming CDK/cyclin complex by phosphorylation leading the dividing cell into next phase of cell cycle. During G1 phase, the predominant cyclin-CDK complexes are cyclin D-Cdk4, 6, cyclin E-Cdk2, cyclin A-Cdk2 during S phase, cyclin A-Cdk1, and cyclin B-Cdk1 during G2/mitotic phases. The control of the G2/M transition is important in all cancers resulting in chromosomal aberrations, but the G1/S transition involves many of the important cell-cycle events that may be altered in breast cancer. G1/S transition involves functions of the oncogenes/tumor suppressors cyclin E, cyclin D1, and p27 [5]. The oncogenic processes do occur by targeting the regulators of G1 phase progression [6]. During the G phase, cells respond to extracellular signals by either going into next division or withdraw from the cycle and thus are arrested in a state (Go). G1 progression is dependent on stimulation by mitogens or growth factors and can be blocked by anti-proliferative cytokines, but cancer cells do not obey these controls. Cancer cells remain in a continuous cycle of cell division by halting maturation and terminal differentiation. Once the cells pass a restriction point late in G1, they do not respond to extracellular growth regulatory signals and commit themselves to the independent program that causes cell division. The cells, which pass through the restriction point G1 and enter into S phase, which is controlled by cyclin-dependent protein kinases (CDKs) that are regulated by cyclins D, E, and A, are committed to divide.

Cyclin D acts as growth factor regulator in response to extracellular signals in the cell cycle. The activity of Cyclin D depends on mitogenic stimulation upon binding with CDK4 and CDK6. Once bound, the catalytic activity of this complex is maximum in G1-S phase transition, but withdrawal of mitogen causes stoppage of cyclin D synthesis, and thus, the D cyclins holoenzyme activities decay rapidly, and the cells exit the cycle [7]. So, if cyclin DI-dependent kinase activity is lost before the restriction point, it prevents cells from entering S phase [8]. To pass through first check point – G1 phase that occurs in normal cell cycle, cyclin D-dependent kinases should phosphorylate protein retinoblastoma tumor suppressor protein (RB) [9]. As the hyper-phosphorylated RB gets dissociated from E2f, DP1, RB complex will result in the activation of E2F genes and leads to transcription of several genes such as cyclin E, cyclin A, and DNA polymerase. RB and other RB-like proteins (pI30, P107), which regulate gene expression which in turn are regulated by a family of heterodimeric transcriptional regulator E2Fs [10], which can transactivate genes and are required for S phase entry [11]. INK4 proteins inhibit (inhibitors of CDK4 and CDK6 INK4 proteins can directly block cyclin D-dependent kinase activity and cause G1 phase arrest) cyclin D-dependent kinases that phosphorylate RB. RB pathway does not functioning normal, which is feature of cancer cells [12]. The RB is inactivated by phosphorylation or by DNA damage; RB gene causes shrinking of G1 phase, and cell size is decreased. The mitogens and other signals required for cell are still present [13]. As the RB negative cells have few requirements for growth factors, these factors in addition to RB phosphorylation work for restriction point control [14]. As the cell cycle proceeds, the cyclin A- and cyclin B-dependent kinases keep RB in its hyper-phosphorylated state. RB is not dephosphorylated until mitosis is completed and again renters the GI phase or Go. The activity of cyclin A synthesis occurs later in GI and is important for the G1-S transition, as blockage of cyclin A function in cells can also block S phase entry. For cell cycle progression, the inactivation of cyclin E and E2F is important when the cell enters S phase [15]. Cyclin B, B-cdc2 complex leads to stimulation of nuclear envelope and initiation of prophase, but its deactivation leads the cell to exit mitosis [16].

2. Drug resistance

Hindrance in treating cancer patient mainly occurs by drug resistance [17]. Targeted therapies on breast cancer depend on the type of receptor being implicated by the expression of estrogen receptor (ER), progesterone receptor (PR), and overexpression of Her2/neu [17]. The therapeutic agents given in such cases, which eventually develop resistance as an acquired drug resistance, are clinically bigger challenge to treat. Thus, patient's resistant to chemotherapy has poor prognosis and overall poor survival [18].

2.1 Cell cycle regulation in tamoxifen-resistant breast cancers

The main drug given to patients expressing estrogen receptor is tamoxifen, which is the first therapeutic agent for the estrogen or progesterone receptor expressing breast cancers, mostly in premenopausal women with or without conventional chemotherapeutic agents [19]. The estrogen receptor (ER) induction occurs during G0/G1 phase in MCF-7 cells and breast cancer cells [19]. In the late S-phase, a rapid increase in ER has been reported [19]. A tamoxifen-resistant phenotype was developed by long-term exposure of MCF-7 xenografts to tamoxifen resulted in an altered expression of ER during the G0/G1 phase [19]. It has been shown that tamoxifen-resistant MCF-7 cells express higher levels of cell cycle regulators cyclin E1 and CDK2 than parental cells [20]. It has been shown that cyclins E1 and E2 were overexpressed in the tamoxifen-resistant cells when compared with parental MCF-7 cells [20]. TAMR cells may be dependent on cyclin E more than MCF-7C, which indicates that CDK2 is inhibited and is a potential therapeutic marker in endocrine-resistant breast cancer [20]. Cyclin E2 downregulation is required for anti-estrogen inhibition of cell proliferation; cyclin E2 overexpression is associated with endocrine resistance in breast cancer providing reason for deregulation of the cell cycle in endocrine resistance [21–24].

3. Genes associated with breast cancer development and its progression

There are various genes associated with breast cancer, and how these respond to different treatments are mentioned as follows:

3.1 EGFR

Epidermal growth factor receptor EGFR (ERBB1 or HER1) is from ERBB family of cell-surface receptor tyrosine kinases including HER2, also known as NEU or ERBB2 [25, 26]. The epidermal growth factor receptor family consists of four cell surface receptors; EGF receptor also called as HER1, HER2 or neu, HER3, and HER4. Epithelial growth factor binds to the receptor and stimulates homo/hetero dimerization of receptor with other ERBB member like HER2, receptor phosphorylation, which makes binding sites available for cytosolic proteins containing *src* homology 2 (SH2) domains [27]. EGFR growth factors cause activation of downstream effectors such as RAS-RAF-MEK-ERK-MAPK and PI3K-AKT-mTOR pathway. PI3K-AKT-mTOR sources irreversible entry of the cell in S phase of cell cycle resulting in cell proliferation [28]. There are various EGFR ligands such as transforming growth factor-α (TGF-α), amphiregulin, epigen, betacellulin, heparin-binding EGF, and epiregulin [29]. EGFR has an important involvement in cellular differentiation, motility, survival, and tissue development [30]. There are many copies of the EGFR gene in some of the breast cancer cells termed as EGFR amplification, which effects on behavior and response of cancer cell. There are other EGFR-positive cancers like colon cancer, which respond to medicines that target EGFR-positive cancers [31]. In a clinical study, there was an increase in EGFR gene copy number in about 6% of breast cancers and protein overexpression in

7% of breast cancers [32]. The study also showed that increased EGFR gene copy number changes, and protein overexpression was seen mostly in ER negative, PR negative, and HER2 negative (triple negative) cases with three exceptions that are HER2-positive cases in total of 175 cases (reference). The study was similar to that of gene expression profiling studies, which have identified EGFR expression mainly in basal-like breast carcinomas (reference). There was another subtype of breast carcinoma that showed an increase in EGFR copy number, or EGFR protein expression is the heterogeneous category of metaplastic carcinoma. These tumors are subtypes called as basal-like breast carcinomas [33] and were seen in 47 metaplastic breast carcinomas in which EGFR protein overexpression was in 32 cases, but gene amplification (as >5 EGFR gene copy number) was seen only in 11 of these 32 (34%) cases [33]. There are other studies that have shown that EGFR gene amplification and EGFR protein overexpression in various organ systems have found similarity in approximately 50% cases [34]. EGFR protein expression is the result of multiple genomic processes of which EGFR gene amplification is only one of them [34]. EGFR protein expression is seen in breast carcinoma, which is mostly triple negative, and there exists a relation between EGFR gene copy number and protein expression, but relation is not as strong as seen with HER2 [34]. The therapeutic use of EGFR as a responsive marker in breast carcinoma is being studied and needs to identify breast cancer patients that will respond to EGFR-related therapies. A new mechanism-based inhibitors and combination therapies are being worked to overcome therapeutic resistance in tumors [34–36].

3.2 HER2

HER2 gene is amplified in breast cancers by about 20% categorized as HER2-positive breast cancers [37], the extra HER2 protein leads to increase in activation of signal pathway, which results in uncontrolled growth and occurrence of cancer. Breast tumors having HER2 overexpressed proteins are more aggressive than other breast tumors [37]. This results in poorer prognosis in patients and decreased survival rate compared with patients whose tumors do not overexpress HER2 [37]. The inhibition of HER2 signaling will provide a tool to reduce breast cancer. Monoclonal antibodies like lapatinib are used to inhibit the signaling [37]. Herceptin (trastuzumab) is also a monoclonal antibody binding to HER2 [37]. This stops receptor from activating the signaling pathways, which is responsible for proliferation and survival of breast cancer cells [37]. Herceptin also causes inhibition of cancer cell growth by activating an immune response, which will damage nearby cells [37]. It is used to treat breast cancer only in tumor overexpressing HER2 with at least one high risk like estrogen receptor or progesterone receptor negative, pathologic tumor size greater than 2 cm, Grades 2–3, age less than 35 years [37]. Herceptin is used in combination with paclitaxel for first-line treatment of HER2-overexpressing metastatic breast cancer [37].

And as a single agent for treatment of HER2-overexpressing breast cancer in patients who have received one or more chemotherapy regimens for metastatic disease [33, 37, 38].

3.3 HSP27

Heat shock protein 27 (HSP27) is the small molecular weight heat shock protein (HSP) family (12–43 kDa). HSP27 and different members of small HSP family possess a conserved c-terminal domain, the α-crystallin domain, which is similar to the vertebrate eye lens α-crystallin [39]. HSP27 was originally characterized in response to heat shock as a protein chaperone making proper refolding of damaged proteins [40].

It has been seen that HSP27 protein also responds to cellular stress such as oxidative stress and chemical stress. HSP27 is a protein, which functions as a protein chaperone, as an antioxidant helps in inhibition of apoptosis and actin cytoskeletal remodeling, regulation of cell development, cell differentiation, and signal transduction [41]. The oligomerization state of HSP27 is due to chaperone activity as the aggregates of large oligomers have high chaperone activity, whereas dimers have no chaperone activity. Large aggregates are formed under heat shock [40]. Hsp27 occurs in all cell types, mostly of muscle cells. It is located mainly not only in the cytosol but also in the perinuclear region, endoplasmic reticulum, and nucleus. It is overexpressed during cell differentiation and development. It has an essential role in the differentiation of tissues [41].

HSP27 functions as an antioxidant during oxidative stress, which lowers the levels of reactive oxygen species (ROS) by increasing the levels of intracellular glutathione and lowering the levels of intracellular iron [40, 42]. During chemical stress, protein acts as an anti-apoptotic agent through mitochondrial-dependent and -independent pathways of apoptosis [43]. During Fas-FasL-mediated apoptosis, HSP27 binds DAXX and stops the binding of Ask1 by DAXX [43]. HSP27 also interplays with Bax and cytochrome c stopping mitochondrial-dependent apoptosis [43]. HSP27 is mostly useful in protection from programmed cell death by inhibition of caspase-dependent apoptosis [43]. The anti-apoptotic properties of HSP27, which occur due to chemical stress, have been useful in chemotherapies such as doxorubicin and gemcitabine [44, 45]. HSP27 regulates actin cytoskeletal dynamics during heat shock and stress conditions, promotes both actin polymerization, and concerts as an actin capping protein. The upregulation of HSP27 is a biomarker acting in some of the disease subsequently, a cell safeguards itself from death or reduces oxidative stress by the help of HSP27 [46].

In vitro studies have shown that HSP27 acts as an ATP-independent chaperone by inhibiting protein aggregation and stabilizing partially denatured proteins, which ensures refolding by the Hsp70-complex [46]. It also preserves the focal contacts fixed at the cell membrane [46]. The main function of Hsp27 is to provide thermo tolerance in vivo, cytoprotection, and support of cell survival under stress conditions [46]. Another function of Hsp27 is the activation of the proteasome. It speeds up the degradation of irreversibly denatured proteins and junk proteins by binding to ubiquitinated proteins and to the 26S proteasome [46]. Hsp27 enhances the activation of the NF-κB pathway that controls a lot of processes, such as cell growth and inflammatory and stress responses [47]. Various reports have confirmed that cytoprotective properties of Hsp27 have been attributed to its ability to modulate reactive oxygen species production and to raise glutathione levels [47]. Hsp27 is known to play a role in the process of cell differentiation [47].

Hsp27 expression is varied in several cells such as Ehrlich ascites cells, embryonic stem cells, normal B cells, B-lymphoma cells, osteoblasts, keratinocytes, and neurons [47]. The upregulation of Hsp27 relates with the rate of phosphorylation and with an increase in large oligomers [48]. It is possible that Hsp27 plays a crucial role in the termination of growth [40].

3.4 HSP27 in breast cancer

Tumor cells show an increase in transcription of heat shock proteins (HSPs) due to loss of p53 functions and increased expression of proto-oncogenes such as HER and c-Myc, which is important for tumorigenesis [49]. Cellular protection and protein folding being the entailed function of HSPs are operative during oncogenesis [49]. Since tumor cell growth and survival are enabled by the increased expression of HSPs. HSP27 is mostly the important heat shock protein involved in protection from programmed cell death by inhibiting caspase-dependent apoptosis [45]. Since HSP27 has been associated with poor prognosis in many types of cancers such as gastric, liver, and prostate carcinoma, osteosarcoma, rectal, lung, and breast cancer [45]. HSP27 has been reported to play an important drug resistance in breast cancer, and some other cancers, HSPs, are involved in immune tolerance by cancer cells and are important targets for cancer therapy process [50]. A study done by Langer et al. in 2008 found that the protein expression profiles in patients with esophageal adenocarcinomas from two groups have shown as responsive and nonresponsive to neo-adjuvant platin and 5-fluorouracil based chemotherapy. The study showed that low HSP27 expression has a correlation with nonresponsiveness to the chemotherapy application [49]. It shows that low levels of HSP27 expression are associated with a negative outcome in cancer. HSP27 levels were studied in patients having colon or rectal cancer [49]. It showed that high HSP27 expression level results in incomplete resection margins in rectal cancer and poor survival.

HSP27 expression was not having any role in survival of colon cancer group but was related to poor survival in the rectal cancer group [49]. The metastatic breast cancer cell lines, which overexpress Her2 and are resistant to Herceptin (SK-BR3 HR), also overexpress HSP27 [49]. The downregulation of HSP27 protein levels was shown by transfecting with siRNA, where Herceptin resistance was also reduced in SK-BR3-HR cells [49]. HSP27 could form a complex with Her2, resulting in a potential mechanism by which the protein potentiates [51]. Her2 overexpressing breast cancer tumors have showed increased expression of phosphorylated HSP27, particularly at serine 78 [51, 52].

3.5 H2AX (H2A histone family, member X)

Histone H2A is programmed by a gene H2AFX (H2A histone family, member X), as H2A is one of the four core histones of DNA in humans and eukaryotes [53]. H2AX helps in nucleosome formation and in the structure of DNA. DNA known as the most stable material present, whose damage occurs due to ionizing radiation, hypoxia, reactive oxygen species, chemicals, and replication or transcriptional errors, which causes activation of DNA repair pathway [53]. Different materials can cause different types of damage in DNA-like double stranded breaks (DSBs), where both DNA strands have been cleaved [53]. If the damage occurred is not repaired, DSBs are lethal for the cell. DNA damage leads to an activation of the DNA damage repair pathway, phosphorylation of histone H2AX on serine 139. Activation of downstream pathway is done by the kinases of the PI3 family (ataxia telangiectasia mutated, ATR, and DNA-PKcs), which are responsible for this phosphorylation, especially ATM. γ-H2AX enrolls other factors, for example, 53BP1, BRCA1, MDC1, and the MRE11-RAD50-NBS1 (MRN) complex to sites of damage [53]. The DSBs, which are not repaired due to irradiation induced γ-H2AX foci, have been used in tumors as a biomarker for sensitivity to radiotherapy [54]. Endogenous γ-H2AX foci are present in normal primary human cells and tissues [54]. In tumor cells, phosphorylated H2AX exists in different levels in the absence of exogenously DSBs [54]. Instability of chromosomes occurs in cells having more endogenous foci [41]. The colocalization of these endogenous foci in association with other DNA repair factors, for example, 53BP1, MRN complex shows that DNA repair occurs at these sites [54]. The endogenous expression of γ-H2AX is present not only in tumor cell lines but also in cancer tissues and in their precursor lesions, which gives an insight into activated DNA damage repair in tumorigenesis [55]. The endogenous expression of DNA damage response factors is also due to damaged, shortened telomeres and hypoxia [56, 57].

Constitutive γ-H2AX expression is higher in triple negative and in BRCA1 and p53-mutated breast cancer cell lines, which makes a relation between endogenous γ-H2AX expression and 53BP1 expression in breast cancer tissue [55]. Other studies have also supported that triple negative breast cancers are having more endogenous γ-H2AX expression and have higher chances of carrying errors in components of the DNA damage repair pathway [55, 57]. Higher occurrence of γ-H2AX positive is present in basal like and triple negative tumors that are BRCA1 mutation carriers. So, the breast cancer patients having high endogenous γ-H2AX or 53BP1 expression showed a subset of triple negative tumors with poor prognosis. The expression of endogenous γ-H2AX in cancers is due to telomeres (protective structures that form the chromosome ends in eukaryotes) [57].

Cell having DNA damaged after duplication of DNA results in shortened telomeres after every cell cycle, so in precancerous event, there occurs shortening of telomeres and activation of telomerase, an enzyme necessary for telomere lengthening [58]. Telomere shortening in normal process is an action for replication arrest and replicative senescence, but in the absence of a telomeric structure, chromosome ends are not stable and are likely either to undergo degradation, combining with other chromosomes resulting in genomic instability or having DNA double-stranded breaks [58]. A good number of endogenous γ-H2AX foci present, which do not have actual double-stranded breaks, are in fact uncapped telomeres, but the DNA damage and phosphorylation of H2AX at these sites occur due to nonfunctioning of telomere [58]. Telomere-associated chromosomal rearrangements may lead to a tumor phenotype with the associated immortality and replicative potential without any barrier [58, 59].

4. PARP poly ADP ribose polymerase

4.1 PARP in normal cells

PARP1 (protein) repairs single-strand breaks of DNA in a normal cell when it is damaged or mutated, and the cell survives when its DNA repaired, but sometimes when the DNA repair mechanism fails, the cell undergoes suicidal apoptotic process, subsequently that the damaged DNA is not passed to progeny cells [60]. When DNA is damaged or requires repair, one of the proteins, which is involved in repairing damaged DNA, is poly (ADP ribose) polymerase 1, or PARP1 moves at the site of damage, gets activated, and enables various DNA repair proteins to repair the broken strand of DNA, but if the breaks in DNA are not repaired until DNA replication occurs, then the replication itself causes double-strand breaks to form [60]. Inhibition of PARP1 is done by number of drugs, which causes double-strand breaks. Tumors having BRCA1, BRCA2, or PALB2 mutations where repair is not done, the double-strand breaks cannot be repaired causing death of cells [61]. In normal cells, DNA replication is not as frequent as in cancer cells, and they also do not have mutated BRCA1 or BRCA2 but have homologous repair mechanism, which makes them to survive the inhibition of PARP [61]. There are cancer cells that lack the tumor suppressor PTEN and maybe sensitive to PARP inhibitors because of downregulation of Rad51, a critical homologous recombination component [33]. A study has shown that PARP inhibitors may also be effective against PTEN-defective tumors like prostate cancers. Most of the tumors are sensitive to PARP inhibitors [61].

4.2 PARP in breast cancer cells

DNA damage in dividing cells or tumor cells is caused mainly by the chemotherapeutic drugs and radiation therapy, but if PARP repairs the damage caused by these agents, the tumor cells survive and grow.

4.3 Inhibiting PARP: mechanism of action

The preclinical studies have shown that standard therapies alone are not as effective as in combination with PARP inhibitors; they are used in cancer cells, which make protein unable to function during chemotherapy, which results in apoptosis of the cell where DNA is unrepaired [61]. In inherent DNA repair defects, such as breast tumors with mutations in the DNA repair proteins BRCA1 or BRCA2, PARP inhibitors are effective as single agents, and they undergo an arrest of the cell cycle and apoptosis on exposure to PARP inhibitors, whereas cells with normal BRCA proteins survive and continue to grow [61]. It has also been predicted that cancer cells with BRCA1 or BRCA mutations are more sensitive to PARP inhibitors to undergo growth arrest and apoptosis than cells with normal BRCA1 or BRCA2 [61]. This occurs due to combination of PARP and loss of BRCA1 or BRCA2 function causing inactivation of two major forms of DNA repair [61], and the damaged cells are not able to maintain the integrity of their genome and become more prone to apoptosis [37, 38, 62].

Function of PARP inhibitors is to block PARP enzyme activity, which stops the repair of DNA damage and causes the cell death [62]. In one of a clinical study that has shown the PARP inhibitors localize PARP proteins near the site of DNA damage, which suggests its role in antitumor activity [62]. The PARP inhibitors are able to trap PARP proteins on damaged DNA, and this function varies among inhibitors, for example, PARP family of proteins in humans includes PARP1 and PARP2, which are used in binding of DNA and protein repair action [63]. DNA damage causes activation of these proteins; they recruit other proteins that are actually involved in repairing DNA [63]. In normal condition, PARP1 and PARP2 are released from DNA when the repair mechanism is in process [64]. The study shows that when they are attached to PARP inhibitors, PARP1 and PARP2 become trapped on DNA [38]. The trapped PARP-DNA complexes are more harmful to cells than the single-strand DNA breaks, which are not repaired that accumulate in the absence of PARP activity resulting in harmful action of PARP inhibitors [38, 62]. There may be two classes of PARP inhibitors, catalytic inhibitors that block PARP enzyme activity and do not trap PARP proteins on DNA and dual inhibitors that both inhibit PARP enzyme activity and act as PARP poison [38, 63, 64]. Various PARP inhibitors are used in clinical trials as shown in **Table 1**.

4.4 PARP in combination with chemotherapy

A number of studies have been done to see the toxicity with PARP inhibitors as monotherapy in tumors with homologous recombination defects and have been compared with chemotherapy [68]. Moreover, in some studies, combination of

PARP inhibitors	Cancer types	References
BMN-673	BRCA mutated breast cancer	[62]
Olaparib	Breast, ovarian, and colorectal cancer	[15]
Veliparib	Melanoma and breast cancer	[65]
CEP 9722	Non-small-cell lung cancer	[66]
MK 4827	Inhibitor of PARP1 and PARP2	[67]
3-aminobenzamide	PARP inhibitor	[67]
Rucaparib	Metastatic breast and ovarian cancer	[15]

Table 1.
PARP inhibitors used in various types of cancers.

PARP inhibitors is used in combination with chemotherapy. PARP inhibitors as known can act as chemo sensitizing agents [68]. The resistance to chemotherapy drugs occurs when PARP repairs the DNA damage caused by these agents, for example, temozolomide is an alkylating agent, which causes DNA damage in which PARP inhibitors act as potential anticancer agents [68].

4.5 PARP in combination with radiotherapy

Radiotherapy causes DNA strand breaks leading to DNA damage and cell death; however, it kills all of the targeted cells, having side effects [68]. Combining radiation therapy with PARP inhibitors has been used to overcome the side effects as these inhibitors form double-strand breaks from the single-strand breaks generated by the radiotherapy in tumor tissue with BRCA1 or BRCA2 mutations. In such cases, the combinatorial therapy leads to better and efficient response with less dose of radiation [68].

5. ROS

Reactive oxygen species (ROS) are reactive molecules containing oxygen [69]. These molecules are formed when a chemical reaction takes place, for example, between oxygen ions and peroxides [69]. ROS plays an important role in cell signaling and homeostasis, due to environmental stress like UV or heat exposure, and ROS levels are increased, which damage cell structure and its function [69].

5.1 ROS in cancer

ROS being secondary messengers in cell signaling are required for various biological processes in normal cells; any dysfunction in redox balance results in human cancers [27]. ROS are increased mostly in cancer cells when oncogenes are activated, and there is lack of blood supply, which initiates progression and metastasis of cancer [27]. ROS levels decide the difference between tumor and nontumor cells [27]. Generation and elimination of ROS at the same time in the system are the expenditure to operate regulatory pathways in a normal physiological condition of cell, and this process is balanced by scavenging system [27]. When oxidative stress occurs, ROS are generated more, which cause carboxylation of cellular proteins, peroxidation of lipids, and DNA damage leading to dysfunction of cell resulting in carcinogenesis, while in cancer cells, ROS stress causes increased metabolism and mitochondrial dysfunction [27]. Consequently, ROS have dual function, on one side, it helps in survival of cancer cell, as cell cycle progression, which is regulated by growth factors via receptor tyrosine kinase activation and chronic inflammation, is regulated by ROS [62]. On an altered side, an increase in ROS level suppresses tumor growth by activating cell cycle inhibitors, which induces cell death and senescence by damaging macromolecules [62]. This dual mechanism helps in chemotherapy and radiotherapy, where cancer cells are killed by ROS stress. The cancer cells are able to differentiate between ROS as survival or apoptotic signal because of the dosage, duration, type, and site of ROS production [66]. ROS is used for survival of cancer cells in moderate level and kills cancer cells in excessive level [66]. Effects of ROS are maintained by cell metabolism by producing antioxidant molecules such as reduced glutathione (GSH) and thioredoxin (TRX), which depend on the reducing power of NADPH to maintain their function (reference) [27]. Sometimes tumor cells overproduce ROS because the NADPH oxidase is regulated by the GTPase Rac1, which is a downstream of proto-oncogene Ras [27].

ROS when associated with cancer activate various transcription factors such as nuclear factor kappa-light-chain-enhancer of activated B cells—NF-κB, activator protein-1—AP-1, hypoxia-inducible factor-1α, and signal transducer and activator of transcription 3—STAT3, which cause protein expression for inflammation, cell transformation, tumor cell survival and proliferation and invasion, angiogenesis, and metastasis (reference). ROS also control the expression of different tumor suppressor genes such as p53, retinoblastoma gene (Rb), and phosphatase and tensin homolog (PTEN) [70–73].

The several causes for oxidative stress in breast cancer cells are as follows:

- Thymidine phosphorylase induction in cancer cells is caused by oxidative stress, an enzyme that is overexpressed in breast cancer. Thymidine phosphorylase catabolizes thymidine to thymine and 2-deoxy-D-ribose-1-phosphate, which is a very powerful reducing sugar that rapidly glycates proteins, generating oxygen radicals within the cancer cell [74].

- Glucose deprivation and hypoxia is caused by continuously usage of blood supply which causes increased cellular oxidative stress in MCF-7 breast cancer cell line but does not increase in nontransformed cell line, reason being glucose deprivation depletes intracellular pyruvate in breast cancer cell, which prevents the decomposition of endogenous oxygen radicals [75]. Study done [76] supports that breast tumor increases its blood supply, leading to glucose deprivation and hypoxia thus causing glucose deprivation, which rapidly induces cellular oxidative stress within the MCF-7 breast carcinoma cell line, although it does not cause oxidative stress in nontransformed cell lines [75]. Cancer cells like breast cancer cells cause increase in blood vessel development (angiogenesis process), where blood flow causes hypoxia followed by reperfusion, which leads to myocardial infarction leading to generation of ROS which leads to oxidative stress in breast cancer [75].

- Breast tumors are accompanied by macrophage population [75]. Oxygen radicals are produced by macrophages; it causes oxidative stress in murine mammary tumor cells. Also, tumor necrosis factor is secreted by macrophages, which also cause cellular oxidative stress [67, 77].

5.2 Effects of ROS in breast cancer

Increase in mutation rate and tumor progression is caused mainly by ROS in which oxygen radicals cause DNA damage, which result in strand breaks, alterations in guanine and thymine bases, and sister chromatid exchanges [78]. ROS lead to inactivation of tumor suppressor genes in tumor cells and increase expression of proto-oncogenes; thus, genetic instability due to persistent oxidative stress in cancer cell will increase malignancy of the tumor [79]. In vitro ROS cause initiation of growth sensing signaling pathways due to cell proliferation in response to hydrogen peroxide because of activation of mitogen-activated protein kinases (MAPKs), like HeLa cells when treated with hydrogen peroxide lead to activation of all three MAPK pathways, extracellular signal-related protein kinase, c-Jun amino-terminal kinase, and stress-activated protein kinase and p38 [79]. Hyper-phosphorylation of c-Jun by oxidative stress activates activator protein-1 in MCF-7 breast cancer cells, which stimulates proliferation [80]. Multidrug-resistant human breast carcinoma cells lead to activation of extracellular signal-related protein kinase-2 when stressed by glucose deprivation [76]. ROS may also cause stimulation of mitosis by

MAPK-independent mechanisms. Oncogenic Ras causes ROS production by activating Rac1 and NADPH-oxidase. It has been also seen that in Ras-transformed human fibroblasts, ROS control cell cycle progression without the activation of MAPK pathways [81, 82].

5.3 Resistance to therapy

Apoptosis is caused by oxidative stress, which is induced depending on p53 in both mouse and human cells [83]. Resistance to apoptosis is caused by persistent oxidative stress [84], whereas the resistant to cytolysis by hydrogen peroxide may be explained by an upregulation of anti-ROS mechanism in cancer cells. Hydrogen peroxide activates anti-apoptotic Akt (protein kinase B) leading response to chronic oxidative stress that can be used for anticancer therapy though in radiotherapy, photodynamic therapy, and other chemotherapies generating oxygen radicals showing antitumor activity [85]. This is due to the induction of tumor cell apoptosis in response to oxidative stress and oxygen radical prompted DNA damage [85]. This results in persistent oxidative stress within carcinoma cells causes resistance to therapy that is further increased by oxygen radicals leading to an increasing carcinoma cell expression of P-glycoprotein, the multidrug-resistance efflux pump [86].

Angiogenesis, which may be one of the reasons for oxidative stress, leads to tumor growth in blood borne metastasis of breast tumor, where oxygen radicals cause tumor migration causing increased risk of invasion and metastasis by activation of p38 MAPK and subsequent phosphorylation of heat shock protein-27 by p38 MAPK causing changes in actin dynamics [46, 79]. Studies have shown that phosphorylated heat shock protein-27 promotes the migration of MDA-MB-231 breast cancer cells on laminin-5 in vitro [41]. Oxidative stress in breast tumors causes invasion and metastasis by activating MMPs as well as by inhibiting antiproteases. MMP-2 as gelatinase has a major role in breast cancer invasion and metastasis; once its levels are high, there is a poor prognosis in breast cancer patients [87]. Subsequently, MMP-2 is seen more in malignant than in benign breast tumors; therefore, it is ROS, which also activate MMP-2 due to reaction of oxygen radicals with thiol groups within MMP-2 [88]. Oxygen radicals inactivate protease inhibitors, such as α1-proteinase inhibitor and plasminogen activator by oxidation of methionine residues at their active sites [65], leading to protease activation, which increase invasion and metastasis processes, for example, plasminogen activator causes metastasis [65].

Cancer cells synthesizing ROS at a higher level in vitro and tumors in vivo are under persistent oxidative stress, as oxygen radicals lead to a poorer prognosis, antioxidants can be used for therapeutic role in breast cancer [89]. Various research studies have shown that human melanoma cells were transfected with cDNA encoding the antioxidant enzyme manganese superoxide dismutase leading to suppression of malignancy; cells not only lost their ability to form colonies on soft agar but also no longer formed tumors in nude mice [89]. Various anticancer therapies are there, which add to the oxidative stress within breast cancer such as chemotherapeutic agent's doxorubicin, mitomycin C, etoposide, and cisplatin, which are superoxide generating agents [85], radiotherapy, and photodynamic therapy, which generate oxygen radicals within the carcinoma cell, and anti-estrogen tamoxifen used in breast cancer therapy also induces oxidative stress within cancer cells in vitro [90]. Conversion of breast tumors to a tamoxifen-resistant phenotype that has been seen is associated with a progressive shift toward a pro-oxidant environment of cells as a result of oxidative stress [90].

6. P53

P53 protein, a tumor protein present in humans, which is encoded by the TP53 gene (tumor suppressor gene), functions to inhibit proliferation of cells and regulates cell cycle, thereby preventing cancer, also called as the guardian of the genome as it maintains the stability in a cellular process preventing genetic mutation, under normal cellular phenomenon the p53 signaling pathway is in static mode, whereas its activation occurs when there is a cellular stresses like DNA damage or oncogene activation [91, 92]. Post-translational modifications activate P53 protein for DNA binding, transactivating downstream effector genes whose activation depends on the nature of stress and its extent. After oxidative stress transcriptional coactivators, for example, apoptosis stimulating protein of p53 and BRCA1 promotes various cellular processes like apoptosis, other components of signaling pathway which are targeted for genetic and epigenetic changes in breast cancer, for example, activation of MDM2 which acts as a negative feedback regulator of the pathway by promoting the degradation of p53 [93].

6.1 P53 mutations in breast cancer

p53 being activator of apoptosis or cell cycle arrest is generated upon DNA damage, or cellular stress has a major role in cancer as it stimulates genomic stability and anti-angiogenic effects, manages tumor inflammation and immune response, and represses metastases [94]. TP53 is mutated mostly in 50% of all human cancers and in 20–30% of breast cancers with more than 15,000 different mutations, which makes P53 as a potential biomarker for breast cancer [94].

In one of a clinical study, it was studied that in premenopausal women, p53 mutation is associated with ER and PR tumors, but in postmenopausal women having breast cancer, the presence of a p53 mutation is associated with higher body mass index (BMI), higher-grade, and poorly differentiated tumors, so women having tumors as well as p53 mutations had a 2.4-fold increased risk of dying from their disease [53]. In an additional clinical study, it has been shown that TP53 mutated noninflammatory locally advanced breast carcinomas respond to doxorubicin-cyclophosphamide chemotherapy unlike TP53 wild-type tumors, due to senescence in TP53 wild-type tumor cell and in MMTV-Wnt1 mammary tumors, growth arrest and senescent phenotype were stimulated in TP53 WT tumors following doxorubicin treatment, and there was no apoptosis while the absence of arrest in mutant tumors caused aberrant mitosis, cell death, and a better clinical response [53, 95]. In ER-positive breast tumors, ER represses the p53-mediated apoptotic response induced by DNA damage, but in ER-negative TP53 mutated breast cancers, accumulation of genetic abnormalities may lead to mitotic catastrophe and better response [95].

6.2 P53 and chemotherapy

Previous clinical studies done on breast cancer patients [96] have seen that ER (+) tumors (mostly TP53 wild type) are mostly resistant to chemotherapy, while ER (−) tumors (mostly a TP53 mutated) are more chemo sensitive, but in another study, it was found that there was no association shown in sensitivity to classical doses of taxane-based therapy and mutated TP53 in breast tumor [97]. TP53 wild-type tumor cells in human breast xenograft models have the presence of senescence in breast cancers in response to the treatment [95] senescence induction and cell cycle arrest in TP53 wild type tumors showed tumor proliferation after the end of treatment while genetic abnormalities and mitotic catastrophe would occur with further response to treatment in TP53 mutated tumors, which was also seen in MMTV-Wnt1 mammary tumors [95]. It has also been seen that growth arrest and senescent phenotype and no apoptosis were induced in TP53 wild-type tumors following doxorubicin treatment, while lack of arrest in R-172-H mutant tumors resulted in aberrant mitoses, cell death, and a better clinical response; wild-type tumors or mutant tumors, which were having a wild-type TP53 allele, did not show apoptosis and did not lose any volume as did TP53 mutant tumors [98]. In ER (+) breast cancers, it was shown that there is a functional interplay between p53 and ER on a genome wide scale and that ER represses the p53-mediated apoptotic response induced by DNA damage, and distinct TP53 gene signatures are also needed to evaluate prognosis and response to chemotherapy in ER-positive and ER-negative breast cancers [74].

Thus, these clinical findings provide a way how to study p53-mediated response to dose-dense doxorubicin-cyclophosphamide chemotherapy in breast carcinomas in ER (+) TP53 wild-type breast tumors and that ER-induced inhibition of p53 apoptotic response would result in tumor cell senescence and resistance to treatment. However, in ER (−) TP53 mutated breast carcinomas, mostly in those having lost both TP53 alleles, there is an increase in genetic abnormalities that lead to mitotic catastrophe and better response [74].

6.3 P53 and ROS signaling

p53, a tumor suppressor protein being redox active transcription factor, organizes and directs cell function during various stresses that lead to genomic instability, on the other hand, reactive oxygen species (ROS) are products or byproducts generated by cells, which function either as signaling molecules or as cell toxicants (reference). Cellular concentration and distribution of p53 have a different cellular function as ROS act as both up-stream signal that causes p53 activation and downstream factor that results in apoptosis [99], subsequently if ROS level is increased due to oxidative stress in cancer cell, then p53 level may be increased to maintain its stability in the environment [99]. A balance is maintained in cellular concentration between oxidant and antioxidant molecules in normal cells, but when the oxidant part increases or when a disruption of redox signaling occurs, oxidative stress is caused in a redox reaction in the system, which results in damage to DNA, proteins, and lipids through oxidative modification resulting in number of diseases and chemotherapeutic cytotoxicity [15].

The genomic stability is maintained by tumor suppressor protein p53, but when there is a cellular stress like disruption of redox signals, which leads to damage DNA, proteins, and lipids. This tumor suppressor gene maintains transcription of various genes and directs cell for cell cycle arrest, senescence or apoptosis through various activation of target genes, many effector molecules like proteins, noncoding RNAs, for example, myc, Hcas or CSE1L, Hzf and miR-34 which help in selecting transactivation of p53 target genes leading to various cellular responses comes into play [85]. Thus, this oxidative stress is associated with p53-dependent cell cycle arrest, DNA repair, and apoptosis, but a clear understanding of the mechanisms of the interactions between ROS and p53 is still elusive [100].

In unstressed cell or normal cell, P53 has a small half-life and is present in low levels by continuous ubiquitination by Mdm2 COP1 (constitutively photomorphogenic 1) and Pirh2 (p53-induced protein with a RING-H2 domain) and derogation by 26S proteasome, where the physiological levels of p53 have different effects on cellular redox potential either it regulates the pro-oxidant and antioxidant genes or it modulates the cellular metabolism [86, 101].

6.4 Levels of p53 and ROS

Overexpression of p53 transactivates a series of p53-induced genes (PIGs) in which many of these PIGs encode redox active proteins including two ROS-generating enzymes, NQO1-quinone oxido-reductase, PIG3, and proline oxidase (POX, PIG6). The upregulation of these pro-oxidant enzymes will lead to oxidative stress and apoptosis [102, 103]. The pro-oxidant genes, which are upregulated, are BAX, PUMA, and $p66^{shc}$ in which BAX and PUMA stimulate uncoupling of mitochondria, which result in ROS generation from a less efficient electron transport chain, and $P66^{shc}$ is a downstream target of p53, which is present in cytoplasm and is translocated into mitochondria by prolyl isomerase 1 (Pin1) and mitochondrial heat shock protein (mtHsp 70), and pro-apoptotic stimulation of $p66^{shc}$ oxidizes cytochrome c, which produces H_2O_2 and opens mitochondrial permeability transition pore initiating apoptosis, and upregulation of these pro-oxidant enzymes leads to oxidative stress and consequently to apoptosis [102, 103]. More genes have been added to the list of p53-induced pro-oxidant genes, which include BAX, PUMA, and $p66^{Shc}$ of which BAX and PUMA can induce uncoupling of mitochondria, resulting in ROS being generated from a less efficient electron transport chain (ETC) [74, 104]. P53 has a downstream target known as $p66^{Shc}$, which predominantly exists in cytoplasm and is translocated into mitochondria with the help of prolyl isomerase 1 (Pin1) and mitochondrial heat shock protein 70 (mtHsp 70) [105, 106].

Oxidative stress is caused by suppression of antioxidant genes by p53, which increases cellular ROS, for example, MnSOD (manganese superoxide dismutase) is suppressed at the promoter level by p53 activation or overexpression [107].

6.5 Redox regulation of p53

The oxidative stress caused by ROS is related to various p53-mediated cell processes like cell cycle arrest, DNA repair, and apoptosis like increase in generation of ROS in mitochondria when treated with chemotherapeutic agent's results in apoptosis, while oxidative stress in the nucleus causes cells to p53-dependent DNA repair [86, 92]. A number of pathways operating to induce redox and p53 signaling select various p53 target genes that decide the final fate of the cell have been found significant in studies going on cisplatin and ginkgo bilobalide resulted in chemotherapeutics-induced ROS increase C-myc [108]. As soon as C-myc levels increase, it causes suppression of p53 transactivation of $p21^{Cip1}$ blocking cell cycle arrest but does not affect p53-transactivation of the pro-apoptosis gene PUMA leading to apoptosis [108]. The mechanism acts in a same manner as in pathogenic bacterium *Pseudomonas aeruginosa* induced cell death having azurin, a copper-containing redox protein excreted by *Pseudomonas aeruginosa* that binds to p53 and transactivates pro-apoptosis protein Bax resulting in apoptosis [108].

6.6 Redox modification

p53-mediated ROS generation is the most important cellular concentration and subcellular localization function as P53 is a redox sensitive protein, which undergoes redox modification and decides the cell fate on the basis of p53 target genes, and the other factors such as cell type, stress, and intensity of stimuli give an insight into the interaction between ROS and p53 [92, 95].

7. P38-MAP kinase

Response to extracellular stimuli is managed and regulated by intracellular signaling pathways by mitogen-activated protein (MAP) kinase pathways whose members are responsible for signaling cascades, mammalian p38s responses, inflammatory cytokines (TNF-& IL-1), growth factors (CSF-1), ultraviolet irradiation, heat shock, osmotic shock, function in cell differentiation, apoptosis, and autophagy [109]. In general, there are four MAP kinase family subgroups, namely extracellular signal-regulated kinases (ERKs), c-jun N-terminal or stress-activated protein kinases (JNK/SAPK), ERK/big MAP kinase 1 (BMK1), and the p38 group of protein kinases [110]. p38 (p38), a 38-kDa protein when phosphorylated by tyrosine as a responsive protein to LPS stimulation (Han et al. 1993) and its kinases are divided by Thr-Gly-Tyr (TGY) dual phosphorylation motif residues in a TXY (where X is Glu, Pro and Gly in ERKs, JNKs and p38 MAPKs) activation motif by a dual specificity, activation of p38 is not only due to responsive nature on stimulus, but on cell type as well., Insulin signaling is reported to activate p38 in 3T3-L1 adipocytes but downregulates p38 in chick forebrain neuron cells [110].

7.1 p38 in the cell cycle

p38 has been studied in G1, G2, and M phases of the cell cycle [30]. p38 MAPK controls both the G2/M and G1/S cell cycle checkpoint in retort to cellular stress corresponding to DNA damage [30]. It facilitates the cell survival processes and initiation/maintenance of cell cycle checkpoints in retort to particular stimuli [30].

7.2 p38 in senescence and tumor suppression

A number of studies have provided evidence of p38 role in tumorigenesis and senescence [28], when there is a loss of senescence in tumor cells, it has been found that its activation may be decreased in tumors and that its pathway units such as MKK3 and MKK6 are lost resulting in increased proliferation [111].

7.3 p38 role in breast cancer

p38 MAPK in survival of tumor cells functions independently of DNA damage and supplements to metastasis, but this effect is indirectly regulated by p38 MAPK through the mediation of factors responsible for survival or migration of cells, for example, basal stimulation of p38 MAPK in B-cell chronic lymphocytic leukemia (B-CLL) is required for the MMP-9 metalloprotease for survival of these cells grown in the presence of stroma cells [112]. However, *in vivo* studies found that the decreased basal as well as TGFβ1-induced MMP-9 activity in breast cancer cells cause inhibition of p38 MAPK pathway by genetic regulators and pharmacological compounds causing decreased bone metastases [113].

In cell division and cell survival, p38 is studied at checkpoint control [113]. Role of p38 in invasiveness in cultured cell has been seen, which shows that phospho-p38 level is increased in cultured invasive breast cancer cells [95, 114]; increased expression of P38 MAPK in breast cancer has been found in relation to poor prognosis and in invasiveness and metastasis [115]. Overexpression of phosphorylated-P38 MAPK has been seen in ~20% of primary breast carcinomas or in relation to HER2 amplification and tamoxifen resistance and is a potential prognostic marker in breast cancer [116]. Therefore, the role of P38 MAPK in breast cancer cell proliferation remains a subject of study as it has dual function in survival and proliferation depending on the expression of mutant TP53 being present in most ER-breast tumors to develop P38 MAPK inhibitors for the treatment of TP53-mutated, ER-breast cancers, it is expressed at a higher level in ER+ in comparison with ER tumors without post-transductional activation as there was no change in the phosphorylation rate of P38 MAPK [116].

8. Role of tamoxifen resistance in breast cancer

A number of studies have reported the role of P38 MAPK in the resistance of ER+ breast tumors to endocrine therapy [117] and its relation between activated P38 MAPK levels and tamoxifen resistance [114, 118]. It has been reported that P38 MAPK leads to increased ER agonist activity through increased phosphorylation of ER and increased ER signaling through coactivator regulation [76]. There is switch in estrogen receptor signaling from its classical pathway to the AP1-dependent nonclassical pathway upon activation of MAPK by anti-estrogens apart from ER being their main target; thus, the activation of P38 MAPK can reduce the cellular response to endocrine therapy, which has been reported as a biomarker for resistance to endocrine therapy, and its detailed study of expression and its activation in breast tumors may provide a new approach to the resistance of breast cancer to endocrine therapy; also it has been reported that increased phospho-p38 levels have been associated with high expression of EGFR and ErbB2 in tamoxifen-resistant xenografts, where it acts to support nuclear functions of ER [76]. In matched primary and recurrent tamoxifen-resistant tumors (and a parallel study of a mouse xenograft in tamoxifen resistance), a link between phospho-p38 and increased ErbB2 with tamoxifen resistance was found [64, 69, 119, 120]. The graphic illustration of the pathway is displayed in **Figure 1**.

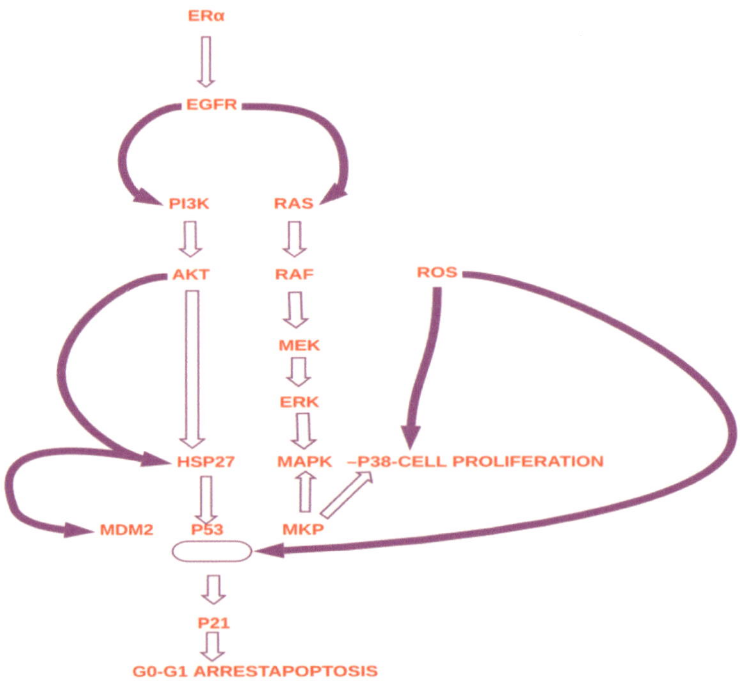

Figure 1.
Signalling pathway affecting estrogen receptor (ER) causing increase in EGFR level leading to cell proliferation during tamoxifen resistivity. P53 is increased during resistance and controls p21 function as well. ROS level is increased causing cell proliferation which in turn decreases Hsp27 and MAPK-P38 activity during stress lead by tamoxifen resistance.

Acknowledgements

The authors acknowledge Sheri Kashmir Institute of Medical Sciences for academic support.

Conflict of interest

The authors declare no conflict of interest.

Author details

Shazia Ali, Mohd Ishaq Dar, Rafiq A. Rather and Dil Afroze*
Advanced Center for Human Genetics, Sher-i-Kashmir Institute of Medical Sciences, Srinagar, Jammu and Kashmir, India

*Address all correspondence to: afrozedil@gmail.com

References

[1] Qin C et al. Estrogen up-regulation of p53Gene expression in MCF-7 breast cancer cells is mediated by calmodulin kinase IV-dependent activation of a nuclear factor Î°B/ CCAAT-binding transcription factor-1 complex. Molecular Endocrinology. 2002;**16**(8):1793-1809

[2] Mendoza-Carrera F et al. Influence of CRP, IL6, and TNFA gene polymorphisms on circulating levels of C-reactive protein in Mexican adolescents. Archives of Medical Research;**41**(6):472-477

[3] Tonetti DA et al. Stable transfection of an estrogen receptor beta cDNA isoform into MDA-MB-231 breast cancer cells. The Journal of Steroid Biochemistry and Molecular Biology. 2003;**87**(1):47-55

[4] Alexis RB, Heldt FS, Zhang T, Bakal C, Bela Nova K, et al. Cell Systems. 2016;**2**:27-37

[5] Marcos MPI, González-Sarmiento R, Laso FJ. Common polymorphisms in interleukin genes (IL4, IL6, IL8 and IL12) are not associated with alcoholic liver disease or alcoholism in Spanish men. Cytokine. 2009;**45**:158-161

[6] Hall JM. The estrogen receptor Â-isoform (ERÂ) of the human estrogen receptor modulates ERÂ transcriptional activity and is a key regulator of the cellular response to estrogens and antiestrogens. Endocrinology. 1999;**140**(12):5566-5578

[7] Sherr JC. G1 phase progression: Cycling on cue. Cell. 1994;**79**(4): 551-555

[8] Baldin VLJ, Marcote MJ, Pagano M, Draetta G. Cyclin D1 is a nuclear protein required for cell cycle progression in G1. Genes & Development. 1993;7(5):812-821

[9] Heinrich PC et al. Principles of interleukin (IL)-6-type cytokine signalling and its regulation. Biochemical Journal. 2003;**374**(1): 1-20

[10] JR N. E2F: A link between the Rb tumor suppressor protein and viral oncoproteins. Science. 1992;**258**(5081):422-429

[11] Mardo Kõivomägi EV, Venta R, Iofik A, Lepiku M, Morgan DO, Loog M. Dynamics of Cdk1 substrate specificity during the cell cycle. Molecular Cell. 2011;**42**(5-4):610-623

[12] Neuhold Barbara Wold L. HLH forced dimers: Tethering MyoD to E47 generates a dominant positive myogenic factor insulated from negative regulation by Id. Cell. 1993;**74**(6):1033-1042

[13] Clarke R et al. Antiestrogen resistance in breast cancer and the role of estrogen receptor signaling. Oncogene. 2003;**22**(47):7316-7339

[14] Novak BTJ, Gyorffy B, Csikasz-Nagy A. Irreversible cell-cycle transitions are due to systems-level feedback. 2007;**9**(7):724-728

[15] Ali F, Hindley C, McDowell G, Deibler R, Jones A, Kirschner M, et al. Cell cycle-regulated multi-site phosphorylation of Neurogenin 2 coordinates cell cycling with differentiation during neurogenesis. 2011;**138**(9):4267-4277

[16] Aster VKAANFJ. Robbins and Cotran Pathologic Basis of Disease, Professional Edition. 8th ed. 2009

[17] Housman G, Byler S, Heerboth S, Lapinska K, Longacre M, Snyder N, et al. Drug resistance in cancer: An overview. Cancers (Basel). 2014;**6**(3): 1769-1792

[18] Pernas S, Sara M. Tolaney HER2-positive breast cancer: New therapeutic frontiers and overcoming resistance. Therapeutic Advances in Medical Oncology. 2019;**11**:1758835919833519

[19] Caponero CHBCSJVR. What is the role of chemotherapy in estrogen receptor-positive, advanced breast cancer? Annals of Oncology. 2009;**20**(7)

[20] Stuart Johnson DNG, Louie TJ, Ruiz NM, Gorbach SL. Sustained clinical response as an endpoint in treatment trials of Clostridium difficile-associated diarrhea. Antimicrobial Agents and Chemotherapy. 2012;**56**(8):4043-4045

[21] Archer SG et al. Expression of ras p21, p53 and c-erbB-2 in advanced breast cancer and response to first line hormonal therapy. British Journal of Cancer. 1995;**72**(5):1259-1266

[22] Varma H, Conrad SE. Reversal of an antiestrogen-mediated cell cycle arrest of MCF-7 cells by viral tumor antigens requires the retinoblastoma protein-binding domain. Oncogene. 2000;**19**(41):4746-4753

[23] Prall OWJ et al. Estrogen-induced activation of Cdk4 and Cdk2 during G1-S phase progression is accompanied by increased cyclin D1 expression and decreased cyclin-dependent kinase inhibitor association with cyclin E-Cdk2. Journal of Biological Chemistry. 1997;**272**(16):10882-10894

[24] Manna S, Holz MK. Tamoxifen action in ER-negative breast cancer. Signal Transduction Insights. 2016;**5**:1-7

[25] Ghayad SE et al. Endocrine resistance associated with activated ErbB system in breast cancer cells is reversed by inhibiting MAPK or PI3K/Akt signaling pathways. International Journal of Cancer;**126**(2):545-562

[26] Fan P et al. Long-term treatment with tamoxifen facilitates translocation of estrogen receptor Â out of the nucleus and enhances its interaction with EGFR in MCF-7 breast cancer cells. Cancer Research. 2007;**67**(3):1352-1360

[27] Becker KA et al. Estrogen and progesterone regulate radiation-induced p53 activity in mammary epithelium through TGF-Î^{2}-dependent pathways. Oncogene. 2005;**24**(42):6345-6353

[28] Ciardiello FTG. EGFR antagonists in cancer treatment. The New England Journal of Medicine. 2008;**358**(11): 1160-1174

[29] Mitsudomi TMS, Yatabe Y, Negoro S, Okamoto I, Tsurutani J, Seto T, et al. Gefitinib versus cisplatin plus docetaxel in patients with non-small-cell lung cancer harbouring mutations of the epidermal growth factor receptor (WJTOG3405): An open label, randomised phase 3 trial. The Lancet Oncology. 2010;**11**(2):121-128

[30] Wang Z et al. Identification, cloning, and expression of human estrogen receptor-Î±36, a novel variant of human estrogen receptor-Î±66. Biochemical and Biophysical Research Communications. 2005;**336**(4):1023-1027

[31] Predicting response to endocrine therapy in breast cancer. Pharma. 1975;**12**(1):11

[32] Fernandez DCBR, Hewitt SM, Levin IW. Infrared spectroscopic imaging for histopathologic recognition. Nature Biotechnology. 2005;**23**(4):469-474

[33] Kaufman B et al. Trastuzumab plus anastrozole versus anastrozole alone for the treatment of postmenopausal women with human epidermal growth factor receptor 2-positive, hormone receptor-positive metastatic breast cancer: Results from the randomized phase III TAnDEM study. Journal of Clinical Oncology. 2009;**27**(33):5529-5537

[34] Hewitt SC, Couse JF, Korach KS. Estrogen receptor transcription and

transactivation estrogen receptor knockout mice: What their phenotypes reveal about mechanisms of estrogen action. Breast Cancer Research. 2000;**2**(5)

[35] Zakaria Z, Zulkifle MF, Hasan WANW, Azhari AK, Raub SHA, Eswaran J, et al. Epidermal growth factor receptor (EGFR) gene alteration and protein overexpression in Malaysian triple-negative breast cancer (TNBC) cohort. OncoTargets and Therapy. 2019;**12**:7749-7756

[36] Wang E, Jiang Z, Ben-David Y, et al. Molecular stratification within triple-negative breast cancer subtypes. Scientific Reports. 2019;**9**:19107

[37] Bergh J et al. Complete sequencing of the p53 gene provides prognostic information in breast cancer patients, particularly in relation to adjuvant systemic therapy and radiotherapy. Nature Medicine. 1995;**1**(10):1029-1034

[38] Keung MYT, Wu Y, Vadgam JV. PARP inhibitors as a therapeutic agent for homologous recombination deficiency in breast cancers. Journal of Clinical Medicine. 2019;**8**(4):435

[39] Agostini L et al. NALP3 forms an IL-1Î-processing inflammasome with increased activity in muckle-Wells autoinflammatory disorder. Immunity. 2004;**20**(3):319-325

[40] Rogalla T et al. Regulation of Hsp27 oligomerization, chaperone function, and protective activity against oxidative stress/tumor necrosis factor Î± by phosphorylation. Journal of Biological Chemistry. 1999;**274**(27):18947-18956

[41] Vidyasagar A, Wilson NA, Djamali A. Heat shock protein 27 (HSP27): Biomarker of disease and therapeutic target. Fibrogenesis & Tissue Repair. 2012;**5**:7

[42] Rust W et al. Heat shock protein 27 plays two distinct roles in controlling human breast cancer cell migration on Laminin-5. Molecular Cell Biology Research Communications. 1999;**1**(3):196-202

[43] Mehlen P et al. Large unphosphorylated aggregates as the active form of hsp27 which controls intracellular reactive oxygen species and glutathione levels and generates a protection against TNFÎ± in NIH-3T3-ras cells. Biochemical and Biophysical Research Communications. 1997;**241**(1):187-192

[44] Charette SJ, Landry J. The interaction of HSP27 with Daxx identifies a potential regulatory role of HSP27 in Fas-induced apoptosis. Annals of the New York Academy of Sciences. 2006;**926**(1):126-131

[45] Cai D et al. Local and systemic insulin resistance resulting from hepatic activation of IKK-Î² and NF-Î°B. Nature Medicine. 2005;**11**(2):183-190

[46] Landry J, Huot J. 6. Regulation of actin dynamics by stress-activated protein kinase 2 (SAPK2)-dependent phosphorylation of heat-shock protein of 27 kDa (Hsp27). In: Cellular Responses to Stress. Princeton University Press

[47] Parcellier A et al. Small heat shock proteins HSP27 and Î±B-Crystallin: Cytoprotective and oncogenic functions. Antioxidants & Redox Signaling. 2005;**7**(3-4):404-413

[48] Abisambra JF, Jinwal UK, Jones JR, Blair LJ, Koren J, Dickey CA. Exploiting the diversity of the heat-shock protein family for primary and secondary tauopathy therapeutics. Current Neuropharmacology. 2011;**9**(4):623-631

[49] Ciocca DR, Calderwood SK. Heat shock proteins in cancer: Diagnostic, prognostic, predictive, and treatment implications. Cell Stress & Chaperones. 2005;**10**(2):86

[50] Mallerstram E et al. Up-regulation of cell cycle arrest protein BTG2 correlates with increased overall survival in breast cancer, as detected by immunohistochemistry using tissue microarray. BMC Cancer;**10**(1)

[51] Zhang D, Wong L, Koay ESC. Phosphorylation of Ser78 of Hsp27 correlated with HER-2/neu status and lymph node positivity in breast cancer. Molecular Cancer. 2007;**6**(1):52

[52] Chatterjee S, Burns TF. Targeting heat shock proteins in cancer: A promising therapeutic approach. International Journal of Molecular Sciences. 2017;**18**(9):1978

[53] Author index to volume 6. Current Molecular Medicine. 2007;**7**(1):1-4

[54] Day CP, James OFW. Steatohepatitis: A tale of two "hits"? Gastroenterology. 1998;**114**(4):842-845

[55] Bartkova JHZ, Koed K, Krämer A, Tort F, Zieger K, Guldberg P, et al. DNA damage response as a candidate anti-cancer barrier in early human tumorigenesis. Nature. 2005;**14**(434):864-870

[56] Shibata AMD, Arvai AS, Perry J, Harding SM, Genois MM, Maity R, et al. DNA double-strand break repair pathway choice is directed by distinct MRE11 nuclease activities. Molecular Cell. 2014;**9**(53):7-18

[57] Nagelkerke KA, van Kuijk SJA, Sweep FCGJ, Nagtegaal ID, Hoogerbrugge N, Martens JWM, et al. Constitutive expression of γ-H2AX has prognostic relevance in triple negative. Breast Cancer. 2011;**101**(1):39-45

[58] Fagerholm RHB, Tommiska J, Aaltonen K, Vrtel R, Syrjäkoski K, Kallioniemi A, et al. NAD(P)H:quinone oxidoreductase 1 NQO1 2 genotype (P187S) is a strong prognostic and predictive factor in breast cancer. Nature Genetics. 2008;**40**(7):844-853

[59] Fardoun MM, Nassif J, Issa K, Baydoun E, Eid AH, A.i.A.n.C.a.L.i. Disclaimer, Raynaud's phenomenon: A brief review of the underlying mechanisms. Frontiers in Pharmacology. 2016;**7**:438

[60] McGlynn EA, Asch SM, Adams J, Keesey J, Hicks J, DeCristofaro A, et al. The quality of health care delivered to adults in the United States. The New England Journal of Medicine. 2003;**348**:2635-2645

[61] Buisson RDCA, Coulombe Y, Launay H, Cai H, Stasiak AZ, Stasiak A, et al. Cooperation of breast cancer proteins PALB2 and piccolo BRCA2 in stimulating homologous recombination. Nature Structural & Molecular Biology. 2010;**17**(10):1247-1254

[62] Murai JHS, Das BB, Renaud A, Zhang Y, Doroshow JH, Ji J, et al. Trapping of PARP1 and PARP2 by clinical PARP inhibitors. Cancer Research. 2012;**1**(72):5588-5599

[63] Gerratanaa L, Basilea D, et al. Androgen receptor in triple negative breast cancer: A potential target for the targetless subtype. Cancer Treatment Reviews. 2018;**68**:102-110

[64] Wu N, Zhang J, Zhao J, Mu K, Zhang J, Jin Z, et al. The overview of breast cancer: Related signaling pathways, therapeutic targets precision medicine based on tumorigenic signaling pathways for triple negative breast cancer. 2018:4984-4996

[65] Swaim MW, Pizzo SV. Review: Methionine sulfoxide and the oxidative regulation of plasma proteinase inhibitors. Journal of Leukocyte Biology. 1988;**43**(4):365-379

[66] MG. PARP inhibitors stumble in breast cancer. Nature Biotechnology. 2011;**29**(5):373

[67] Claire Y, Wenham J, Claire PGC, Wenham YJ. The role of synovitis in

osteoarthritis. Therapeutic Advances in Musculoskeletal Disease. 2001;**6**(10)

[68] Reilly NM, Novara L, Di Nicolantonio F, Bardelli A. Exploiting DNA repair defects in colorectal cancer. 2019;**03**

[69] Yu Z, Song YB, Cui Y, Fu AQ. Effects of AIF-1 inflammatory factors on the regulation of proliferation of breast cancer cells. Journal of Biological Regulators and Homeostatic Agents. 2019;**33**(4):1085-1095

[70] Takahashi KYS. Induction of pluripotent stem cells from mouse embryonic and adult fibroblast cultures by defined factors. Cell. 2006;**126**(4): 663-676

[71] Meyers CASJ, Bezjak A, Mehta MP, Liebmann J, Illidge T, Kunkler I, et al. Neurocognitive function and progression in patients with brain metastases treated with whole-brain radiation and motexafin gadolinium: Results of a randomized phase III trial. Journal of Clinical Oncology. 2004;**1**(22):157-165

[72] Gupta SCPS, Aggarwal BB. Therapeutic roles of curcumin: Lessons learned from clinical trials. The AAPS Journal. 2013;**15**(1):195-218

[73] Aubrey BJ, Strasser A, Kelly GL. Tumor suppressor functions of the TP53 pathway. Cold Spring Harbor Perspectives in Medicine. 2016;**6**(5): a026062

[74] Bailey ST et al. Estrogen receptor prevents p53-dependent apoptosis in breast cancer. Proceedings of the National Academy of Sciences;**109**(44):18060-18065

[75] Spitz DRSJ, Ridnour LA, Galoforo SS, Lee YJ. Glucose deprivation-induced oxidative stress in human tumor cells. A fundamental defect in metabolism? Annals of the New York Academy of Sciences. 2000;**899**:349-362

[76] Commentaire du Travail, de Lee YJ, et al. Endoscopy;**47**(11):1065

[77] Fraser-Brace V, County SJ, et al. International Law Reports. Cambridge University Press. pp. 217-233

[78] Wiseman H, Halliwell B. Damage to DNA by reactive oxygen and nitrogen species: Role in inflammatory disease and progression to cancer. Biochemical Journal. 1996;**313**(1):17-29

[79] Bose S et al. Allelic loss of chromosome 10q23 is associated with tumor progression in breast carcinomas. Oncogene. 1998;**17**(1):123-127

[80] Schiff R. Cross-talk between estrogen receptor and growth factor pathways as a molecular target for overcoming endocrine resistance. Clinical Cancer Research. 2004;**10**(1):331S-3336S

[81] Irani K et al. Mitogenic signaling mediated by oxidants in Ras-transformed fibroblasts. Science. 1997;**275**(5306):1649-1652

[82] Sarmiento-Salinas FL, Delgado-Magallón A, Montes-Alvarado JB, Ramírez-Ramírez D, Flores-Alonso JC, Cortés-Hernández P, et al. Breast cancer subtypes present a differential production of reactive oxygen species (ROS) and susceptibility to antioxidant treatment. Frontiers in Oncology. 2019;**9**:480

[83] Berger CE et al. p53, a target of estrogen receptor (ER), modulates DNA damage-induced growth suppression in ER-positive breast cancer cells. Journal of Biological Chemistry;**287**(36):30117-30127

[84] Casado P et al. Vincristine regulates the phosphorylation of the antiapoptotic protein HSP27 in breast cancer cells. Cancer Letters. 2007;**247**(2):273-282

[85] Kawahara N et al. Enhanced coexpression of thioredoxin and high mobility group protein 1 genes in

human hepatocellular carcinoma and the possible association with decreased sensitivity to cisplatin. Hepatology Research. 1997;**7**(1):71-71

[86] Ziemann C et al. Reactive oxygen species participate in mdr1b mRNA and P-glycoprotein overexpression in primary rat hepatocyte cultures. Carcinogenesis. 1999;**20**(3):407-414

[87] Duffy MJ et al. Breast Cancer Research. 2000;**2**(4)

[88] Rajagopalan S et al. Reactive oxygen species produced by macrophage-derived foam cells regulate the activity of vascular matrix metalloproteinases in vitro. Implications for atherosclerotic plaque stability. Journal of Clinical Investigation. 1996;**98**(11):2572-2579

[89] Church SL et al. Increased manganese superoxide dismutase expression suppresses the malignant phenotype of human melanoma cells. Proceedings of the National Academy of Sciences. 1993;**90**(7):3113-3117

[90] Ferlini C et al. Tamoxifen induces oxidative stress and apoptosis in oestrogen receptor-negative human cancer cell lines. British Journal of Cancer. 1998;**79**(2):257-263

[91] Ciribilli Y et al. The coordinated P53 and estrogen receptor cis-regulation at an FLT1 promoter SNP is specific to genotoxic stress and estrogenic compound. PLoS One;**5**(4):e10236

[92] Al-Madhoun AS et al. The interaction and cellular localization of HSP27 and ERÎ² are modulated by 17Î²-estradiol and HSP27 phosphorylation. Molecular and Cellular Endocrinology. 2007;**270**(1-2):33-42

[93] Mantovani F, Collavin L, Del Sal G. Mutant p53 as a guardian of the cell. Cell Differentiation. 2019;**26**:199-212

[94] Petitjean A et al. Impact of mutant p53 functional properties onTP53mutation patterns and tumor phenotype: Lessons from recent developments in the IARC TP53 database. Human Mutation. 2007;**28**(6):622-629

[95] Bertheau P et al. p53 in breast cancer subtypes and new insights into response to chemotherapy. The Breast;**22**:S27-S29

[96] Bunz FHP, Torrance C, Waldman T, Zhang Y, Dillehay L, Williams J, et al. Disruption of p53 in human cancer cells alters the responses to therapeutic agent. The Journal of Clinical Investigation. 1999;**104**(3):263s-269s

[97] Lonning P et al. Breast cancer prognostication and prediction in the postgenomic era. Annals of Oncology. 2007;**18**(8):1293-1306

[98] Jackson TA et al. The partial agonist activity of antagonist-occupied steroid receptors is controlled by a novel hinge domain-binding coactivator L7/SPA and the corepressors N-CoR or SMRT. Molecular Endocrinology. 1997;**11**(6):693-705

[99] Liu W et al. Disruption of estrogen receptor 1-p53 interaction in breast tumors: A novel mechanism underlying the anti-tumor effect of radiation therapy. Breast Cancer Research and Treatment. 2008;**115**(1):43-50

[100] Kanagasabai R et al. Forced expression of heat shock protein 27 (HSP27) reverses P-glycoprotein (ABCB1)-mediated drug efflux and MDR1 gene expression in adriamycin-resistant human breast cancer cells. Journal of Biological Chemistry;**286**(38):33289-33300

[101] Dornan DWI, Shimizu H, Arnott D, Frantz GD, Dowd P, O'Rourke K, et al. The ubiquitin ligase COP1 is a critical negative regulator of p53. Nature. 2004;**6**(429):86-92

[102] Polyak. Mathematical Programming. 1997;**76**:265

[103] Rivera A. Groundwater news. Natural Resources Canada/ESS/Scientific and Technical Publishing Services. 2005

[104] Sablina AA et al. The antioxidant function of the p53 tumor suppressor. Nature Medicine. 2005;**11**(12):1306-1313

[105] Trinei M et al. A p53-p66Shc signalling pathway controls intracellular redox status, levels of oxidation-damaged DNA and oxidative stress-induced apoptosis. Oncogene. 2002;**21**(24):3872-3878

[106] Pinton P, Rizzuto R. p66Shc, oxidative stress and aging: Importing a lifespan determinant into mitochondria. Cell Cycle. 2008;**7**(3):304-308

[107] Drane P et al. Reciprocal down-regulation of p53 and SOD2 gene expression-implication in p53 mediated apoptosis. Oncogene. 2001;**20**(4):430-439

[108] Zhou R et al. A role for mitochondria in NLRP3 inflammasome activation. Nature;**469**(7329):221-225

[109] Banin S. Enhanced phos-phorylation of p53 by ATM in response to DNA damage. Science. 1998;**281**(5383):1674-1677

[110] Tyler Zarubin QJ, New L, Han J. Identification of eight genes that are potentially involved in tamoxifensensitivity in breast cancer cells. Cell Research. 2005;**15**(6):439-446

[111] Brancho DTN, Jaeschke A, Ventura JJ, Kelkar N, Tanaka Y, Kyuuma M, et al. Mechanism of p38 MAP kinase activation in vivo. Genes & Development. 2003;**17**(16):1969-1978

[112] White CPAE. Does control of mutant p53 by Mdm2 complicate cancer therapy. Genes & Development. 2008;**22**(10):1259-1264

[113] Wheeler TMSK, Lueck JD, Osborne RJ, Lin X, Dirksen RT, Thornton CA. Reversal of RNA dominance by displacement of protein sequestered on triplet repeat R. Science. 2009;**325**(5938):336-339

[114] Massarweh S et al. Tamoxifen resistance in breast tumors is driven by growth factor receptor signaling with repression of classic estrogen receptor genomic function. Cancer Research. 2008;**68**(3):826-833

[115] Smith LM et al. cJun overexpression in MCF-7 breast cancer cells produces a tumorigenic, invasive and hormone resistant phenotype. Oncogene. 1999;**18**(44):6063-6070

[116] Cancello RHC, Viguerie N, Taleb S, Poitou C, Rouault C, Coupaye M, et al. Reduction of macrophage infiltration and chemoattractant gene expression changes in white adipose tissue of morbidly obese subjects after surgery-induced weight loss. Diabetes. 2005;**54**(8):2277-2286

[117] Martin ECES, Rhodes LV, Antoon JW, Fewell C, Zhu Y, Driver JL, et al. Preferential star strand biogenesis of pre-miR-24-2 targets PKC-alpha and suppresses cell survival in MCF-7 breast cancer cells. Molecular Carcinogenesis. 2014;**53**(1):38-48

[118] Gregory M, Gutierrez M, Chow JW, Tillman MD, McCoy SC, Castellano MV, et al. Resistance training improves gait kinematics in personswith multiple sclerosis. Archives of Physical Medicine and Rehabilitation. 2005;**86**

[119] Hommes DW, Peppelenbosch MP, van Deventer SJH. Mitogen activated protein (MAP) kinase signal transduction pathways and novel anti-inflammatory targets. Gut. 2003;**52**(1):144-151

[120] Soni S, Anand P, Padwad YS. PMAPKINAS E MAPKAPK2: The master regulator of RNA-binding proteins modulates transcript stability and tumor progression. Journal of Experimental & Clinical Cancer Research. 2019;**38**:121

Section 2

Breast Cancer Regulatory Pathways

Chapter 2

A Potential New Mechanism for Bisphenol Molecules to Initiate Breast Cancer through Alteration of Bone Morphogenetic Protein Signaling in Stem Cells and Their Microenvironment

Boris Guyot and Veronique Maguer-Satta

Abstract

Endocrine disruptors interfere with endocrine-mediated regulations of cell or organ functions. Estrogens are one of the main hormones altered by endocrine disruptors like bisphenol A (BPA). Stem cells are active from embryogenesis to late stages of adult life. Their unique properties, such as an extended lifespan and low cycling features, render these cell privileged targets of long-term exposure to numerous factors. Therefore, stem cells are likely to be affected following exposure to endocrine disruptors. One of the major signaling pathways involved in stem cell regulation is the bone morphogenetic protein (BMP) pathway. The BMP pathway is known for its involvement in numerous physiological and pathophysiological processes. Exposure of human mammary stem cells to pollutants such as BPA initiates fundamental changes in stem cells, in particular by altering major elements of BMP signaling, such as receptor expression and localization. Lastly, BPA and its substitute bisphenol S (BPS) have similar impacts on BMP signaling despite their different ER-binding properties, supporting the hypothesis that their biological effects cannot be extrapolated only from their interaction with ERα66. We review recent discoveries in this field and discuss their implications for cancer diagnosis, prevention, and treatment, as well as their relevance for studies on endocrine disruptors.

Keywords: BMP, bisphenol, stem cells, breast cancer, microenvironment, endocrine disruptors, estrogen

1. Introduction

Breast cancer is the most common cancer in women and exhibits important phenotypic and genetic diversities associated with different prognoses. Breast cancer subtypes are clinically classified based on histological appearance and expression of hormone receptors such as estrogen (ER) and progesterone (PR) receptors, as well as on the amplification of the HER2 gene coding for a member of the EGF receptor family [1]. Based on these criteria, four major breast cancer subtypes have been defined: luminal A and luminal B (all ER+), HER+ (that can be either ER– or ER+), and basal-like (ER−) [2, 3]. The most frequent subtype encompasses ER-positive tumors that represent almost 80% of breast cancers. In these tumors, preventing ER activation via hormone therapy is efficient. This can be achieved either by using competitive antagonists of estrogens (e.g., tamoxifen), preventing its binding to and subsequent activation of ER, by using drugs blocking estrogen synthesis (antiaromatase) in postmenopausal women, or by luteinizing hormone-releasing hormone (LHRH) analogs, inhibiting release of female hormones by the ovaries [4].

Breast cancer is a multifactorial disease, and evidences of the involvement of extrinsic factors in the increase of breast cancer risk have been described, such as the environment or lifestyle. Indeed, lack of physical activity, elevated tobacco or alcohol consumption, and the use of contraceptive pills or hormone-replacement therapy (for postmenopausal women) have been shown to increase breast cancer risk [5]. Hormonal status has also been described to play a major role in breast cancer risk. It has been shown that a premature or extensive exposure to endogenous estrogens (due to an early menarche, nulliparity, late age for first full-term pregnancy, or late menopause) increases the risk of breast cancer development.

Several chemical pollutants have been classified as endocrine-disrupting chemicals (EDCs) based on the following definition: "an endocrine disruptor is an exogenous substance or mixture that alters any function(s) of hormone actions and consequently causes adverse health effects in an intact organism, or its progeny, or (sub)populations" [6–11]. Estrogens are one of the main hormones altered by EDCs. Perturbations in estrogen functions have been identified in a wide spectrum of pathologies, including metabolic, bone, and reproductive disorders, as well as breast, endometrial, or ovarian cancers. Therefore, it is important to consider that the mammary gland is exposed throughout life not only to endogenous hormones but also to EDCs, molecules present in the environment and able to mimic these hormones.

Interest in EDCs is growing rapidly, owing notably to their extensive use in manufactured goods and their release in our environment. Among these environmental pollutants, bisphenol molecules are being increasingly studied in breast cancer due to their estrogen-mimetic properties, enabling them to activate estrogen signaling through their binding to the ER, in particular, bisphenol A (BPA) [12, 13]. Despite rising concerns about its safety [14] and progressive restrictions on its use, several million tons of BPA are still produced worldwide.

2. The major effects of bisphenols on BMP signaling and stem cells

2.1 BPA and breast cancer

2.1.1 BPA and estrogen signaling

BPA is an aromatic organic compound used by the plastic industry as a monomer in the synthesis of polycarbonates and epoxy resins. Polycarbonates are found in consumer plastic-like water bottles, food packaging materials, sport equipment or toys, while epoxy resins are used to coat the inside of food or beverage containers. BPA can also be found in thermal paper. BPA monomers from these compounds can be released into the environment by hydrolysis. At the structural level, BPA is a diphenyl compound with two hydroxyl groups in a "para" position rendering it highly similar to synthetic estrogen (diethylstilbestrol). This thus allows BPA to interact with various physiological receptors similar to estrogen, including ERs.

The classical genomic estrogen signaling pathway is triggered by the binding of estrogen to its α or β receptors that act as transcription factors in the nucleus. In the absence of ligands, these receptors are complexed with inhibitory molecules either in the cytoplasm or in the nucleus of the cell. Upon ligand binding, these complexes dissociate resulting in conformational changes that allow DNA binding and recruitment of cofactors to regulate expression of target genes [15]. Both ERα and ERβ are also able to initiate a nongenomic signaling pathway outside of the nucleus depending on their subcellular localization [16]. Moreover, estrogen signaling can also be mediated by other receptors, such as GPR30, EGFR, to list only a few [15, 17].

In line with the current definition of EDCs, BPA was shown to exert its activity by disrupting the estrogen signaling pathway that uses ER as a transcription factor binding to estrogen response element (ERE) sites on DNA [15]. Consequently, estrogen-mimetics (e.g., BPA) were mechanistically thought to primarily act through their binding to ERα66, the main canonical (nuclear) estrogen receptor. This nuclear receptor initiates signaling pathways at the cell membrane and transcriptional responses in the cell nucleus. BPA also upregulates the level of steroid receptor coactivators (SRC-1, SRC-3) and promotes the activity of EREs [18]. However, BPA has also been shown to bind to a number of distinct nuclear and membrane receptors, namely estrogen receptors ERα/β, androgen receptor (AR), G protein-coupled ER (GPER, GPR30), PPAR (especially PPARγ), insulin-like growth factor-1 (IGF1-R) [17, 19, 20]. BPA stimulates the release of EGFR ligands by directly targeting other molecules than ER, like ADAM17 or ADAM10 [21]. Furthermore, the impact of BPA on Ca^{2+} release or ERK signaling has been highlighted in the pancreas [15]. Altogether, these results indicate that BPA, in addition to its effects on the canonical estrogen pathway, is able to perturb numerous physiological processes through estrogen genomic and nongenomic signaling, as well as nonestrogen-related pathways [19, 22]. Importantly, BPA is at the origin of toxic derivatives (chlorinated bisphenols) and is also processed by cellular and biochemical mechanisms to generate a number of different BPA metabolites. All these BPA derivatives have been reported to have similar or higher toxic effects than BPA [19, 20]. In the context of the mammary gland, it is thus of utmost importance to further elucidate how BPA, its derivatives or metabolites, modulate estrogen- or nonestrogen-related signaling. This should improve our understanding of the tumorigenic potential of BPA, firstly in the luminal breast cancer subtype, and subsequently in other tumor types.

2.1.2 BPA involvement in breast cancer

Evidence gathered from studies in experimental models and human populations has already confirmed that EDCs, including BPA, contribute to increased risk of disease [23, 24]. A positive relationship between exposure to BPA and cancer development is reported in the literature [25]. However, whether BPA is actually harmful for human health remains understudied, similar to our understanding of the molecular mechanisms underlying BPA-dependent effects in cancer development.

Given the significant involvement of estrogens in both normal and pathological conditions, EDCs able to interfere with the homeostasis of the estrogen endocrine system are a potential source of several health disorders. In this context, a human population-based study detected a significant increase in serum levels of BPA and established a correlation with breast tissue density measured in mammographies [26]. This finding was attributed to the ability of BPA to increase proliferation of mammary epithelial cells from either normal or breast cancer tissues [27, 28]. Epigenetic data from human tumors or cells exposed to BPA *in vitro* revealed the ability of this EDC to directly induce mammary epithelial cell transformation [29].

Moreover, BPA was correlated with breast cancer patients with high risk profiles and therefore with increased disease relapse [30]. This may be due to the implication of BPA in breast cancer metastasis. This process has traditionally been associated with late stages of cancer development, though a new hypothesis on its origin has progressively emerged suggesting that it could be an inherent mark of tumor cell [31, 32]. Metastatic dissemination is a dynamic process that involves several steps: local invasion of cells from the primary tumor, intravasation leading to dissemination through the blood or lymph, extravasation to invade new tissues, implantation, and finally new tumor growth. Numerous signaling pathways and programs are activated during this process such as epithelial-to-mesenchymal transition (EMT), anoïkis, migration, and proliferation among others (for review: [33, 34]). It has been shown that ER-negative breast cancers are associated with an increased risk of developing metastases [35]. Indeed, these breast cancers express more mesenchymal markers such as vimentin and N-cadherin or EMT-transcription factors that are required for metastatic initiation. Conversely, ER-positive tumors are associated with a more differentiated luminal phenotype, expressing epithelial markers (E-cadherin, ER, FOXA1 for instance). Accordingly, a downregulation of the luminal-specific transcription factor FOXA1 is induced after BPA treatment in triple-negative tumor cell lines, leading to the induction of EMT and increasing cell motility [36]. In this study, BPA treatment was shown to activate the PI3K/AKT pathway, leading to a downregulation of epithelial genes alongside an upregulation of mesenchymal genes. Another study demonstrated that BPA promotes migration and invasion via GPER, which transduces FAK, Src, and ERK2 signaling pathway activation [37]. Promotion of GPER-induced migration by BPA or BPS occurs via different signaling pathways. Indeed, in contrast to BPA, which acts via the FAK/Scr/ERK2 pathway, it has been shown that BPS induces GPER/Hippo-YAP-dependent migration [38]. Effects of BPA, BPS, and BPF on migration and EMT properties of ER-positive tumor cell lines were compared [39]. After treatment, cells lost cell/cell contacts and acquired a fibroblast-like morphology associated with an EMT phenotype. This was further confirmed after analysis of EMT-associated protein expression showing a decrease in E-cadherin and an increase in N-cadherin. Moreover, BPA-, BPS-, and BPF-treated cells displayed a stronger migratory ability. All of these modifications were inhibited after administration of an ER antagonist, demonstrating the ER-dependent effects of these bisphenols [39].

At the mechanistic level, a large number of *in vivo* and *in vitro* studies have highlighted the ability of BPA to disrupt several key signaling pathways that are known to be involved in breast cancer [19, 40]. However, the direct involvement of BPA in breast cancer incidence is difficult to establish and remains controversial [26, 41], owing possibly to the fact that different mechanisms are depicted in either ER-positive or -negative tumors, reflecting the variety of biological effects arising from exposure to BPA [20, 28, 42]. In addition, the combinatorial effects of different pollutants encountered over a life time also complicate these studies. Hence, scientists are faced with a huge challenge in order to formally establish the transforming power of BPA, owing to the different contexts and mechanistic cascades of alterations occurring in the human breast tissue during such long-term exposure.

2.2 BPA target cells

2.2.1 Stem cells in mammary gland

Mammary gland development takes place during embryogenesis and is composed of a rudimentary ductal system blocked until puberty. Then, two master reproductive hormones are secreted, namely estrogens and progesterone.

Estrogens control the growth of ducts from their distal extremity called terminal end buds (TEBs) [43–45], while progesterone is involved in lateral branch development [46, 47]. One of the major hormones involved in mammary gland development is estrogen, mostly produced by the ovaries (but also by other tissues). Estrogens, in combination with other hormones, orchestrate the growth of the ductal system and adipose tissue accumulation during puberty and at further stages of development [43–45].

In adults, the mammary gland is formed of ducts and lobules of secreting luminal epithelial cells surrounded by contractile myoepithelial cells. These epithelial cells are embedded in a stroma mainly formed of fibroblasts and adipocytes that secrete several soluble molecules regulating epithelial cell function and differentiation. Epithelial cells of the mammary gland are generated by mammary stem cells (MaSCs) and the stromal compartment by mesenchymal stem cells (MSCs) [48–51]. During adulthood, the mammary gland undergoes functional and structural changes that alternate between phases of proliferation, differentiation, and apoptosis controlled by cyclic hormonal variations due to the estrous/menstrual cycle modulating the stem cell compartment [52]. However, this postpubertal mammary tree remains immature and only achieves full maturation during pregnancy and lactation. These final steps involve alveogenesis and milk production, which take place mostly under the control of progesterone and prolactin [53, 54]. Studies indicate that estrogens do not directly stimulate proliferation of ER-positive luminal cells but act via a paracrine process [55, 56]. Indeed, estrogen acts on luminal ER/PR-positive cells, leading to the cleavage and liberation of amphiregulin [57, 58], which then affects neighboring ER/PR-negative cells. These ER/PR-negative cells display characteristics of stem cells, in that, their asymmetric division is controlled by growth factors released by stromal cells [59–62]. Conversely, estrogen treatment induces a deficient asymmetric division of a human MaSC cell line (MCF10F) [63]. Ovariectomized mice (or letrozole treated to inhibit endogenous estrogen synthesis and provide a normal stromal and hormonal environment for all other hormones) show a decrease in the ability of MaSCs to repopulate a mammary fat pad and to generate ductal growth and expansion without impacting the size of the MaSCs-enriched subpopulation [52]. Collectively, these studies highlight the importance of the estrogen pathway on MaSC regulation through direct and indirect effects and consequently suggest potential sensitivity of these cells to estrogen-mimetics like BPA. Furthermore, stem cells are a unique category of cells active from embryogenesis up to late stages of human adult life, and are thus more prone to be exposed to EDCs, likely altering their normal functions [64–68].

2.2.2 BPA, stem cells, and breast cancer

It has been shown that exposure to EDCs occurs throughout life and even during embryogenesis, at the stage of mammary gland establishment. For instance, BPA has been detected in urinary samples but also in maternal and fetal plasma, in colostrum, and in placental tissue at birth. Several studies demonstrated that a prenatal exposure to BPA induces changes in fetal mouse mammary gland, in the epithelial as well as stromal compartments, favoring fat pad maturation and increasing the mammary gland susceptibility to carcinogens [69–71]. This is accompanied by transcriptome modifications, in particular, an increase in the expression of genes belonging to the antiapoptotic family, myoepithelial differentiation, and adipogenesis, and a decrease in those involved in cell adhesion [71]. Exposure to BPA at puberty alters the function of MaSCs, leading to the appearance in the regenerated glands of early neoplastic lesions with molecular alterations similar to those detected in early neoplastic breast cancer tissues [72]. In a physiological model in which mice were treated at puberty with BPA, estrogen-dependent transcriptional events were perturbed and the number of terminal end buds was altered in a dose-dependent fashion [27]. *In vitro* exposure of normal human mammary epithelial cells to BPA was shown to induce their proliferation due to the secretion of autocrine growth factors and allow them to generate bigger mammospheres [73]. Treated cells displayed an increase in DNA hypermethylation of tumor suppressor genes, such as Brca1. These data support that BPA can promote early pretumoral stages corroborating findings in normal human breast epithelial cells (MCF-10F) [29, 64]. Indeed, BPA-treated human MaSC lines, such as MCF-10F, increase their expression of genes involved in DNA repair and decrease proapoptotic gene expression [74]. Chronic exposure of MCF10A cells to BPA at doses similar to those measured in contaminated water lead to major MaSC modifications affecting their stem cell properties and regulation [64]. Importantly, BPA treatment increases stem-like features by inducing the expression of ALDH1 and SOX2 genes, a human MaSCs marker and a master regulator of pluripotency in embryonic stem cells, respectively [75]. BPA also perturbs signals involved in human mammary stem cell (ERα66 negative cells) regulation, like the bone morphogenetic protein (BMP) pathway, which has been identified in their transformation [76], partly by changing BMP membrane receptor availability and priming cells to BMP signaling [64]. These data raised the hypothesis that in ER-positive tumors, under tamoxifen treatment and in a BPA-containing environment, some cells could acquire resistance to treatment by a switch in signaling pathway favoring a stem-like phenotype characterized by a decrease in treatment cytotoxicity and a modification of the stoichiometry of the type of ER (e.g., an increase in ERRγ or ERα isoform expression).

Overall, these observations strongly support that MaSCs are directly sensitive to BPA, which could be involved in their transformation and/or treatment escape [27, 72, 74].

2.3 BMP, stem cells, and cancer

2.3.1 BMP and mammary epithelial stem cells

One of the major conserved signaling pathways involved in stem cell regulation from embryogenesis up to adult stages is BMP signaling. There are 21 different soluble BMP molecules that act through serine/threonine kinase BMP receptors (BMPRs). In the context of stem cell regulation, BMP2 and BMP4 are progressively emerging as the most important BMPs. The BMP pathway is involved in numerous physiological and pathological processes [77]. BMPs control MSC regulation, such as lineage specification of adipocytes which are one of the major elements of the mammary gland microenvironment [78–80]. Alterations in BMP signaling have been implicated in metabolic disorders such as obesity in women [81, 82].

During embryogenesis in mice, BMP4 was shown to participate in the early steps of mammary gland development by regulating the dorsoventral axis establishment [83]. The BMP pathway also plays a role in mammary bud formation and outgrowth, as well as in ductal branching morphogenesis initiation. Indeed, BMP4 is expressed in both mesenchymal and epithelial cells of the mammary bud and the use of a BMP4 inhibitor leads to a decrease in bud outgrowth [84]. A link between BMPs and progesterone receptor type A involved in branching morphogenesis during postnatal mammary gland development has also been shown [85]. In addition, BMPs are also involved in the myoepithelial compartmentalization and lumen formation [85]. The knockout of a BMP extracellular antagonist, Twisted, abrogates lumen formation and disorganizes the myoepithelial layer through a decrease in

SMAD1-5-8 phosphorylation and the repression of BMP targets (Msx1, Msx2, and Gata-3) [86]. In human cells, BMP2 regulates luminal epithelial cells by modulating the expression of *GATA-3* and *FOXA1* [76]. Finally, an *in vitro* study using sorted mouse mammary epithelial undifferentiated cells demonstrated the role of BMP signaling in final maturation steps such as lactogenic differentiation [87].

In healthy tissues, epithelial cells, as well as cells within the mammary gland environment (fibroblasts, adipose tissue cells, hematopoietic cells), contribute to the production of soluble BMP2 and BMP4 molecules [76], while distinct subpopulations of normal mammary epithelial cells sorted according to CD10 and EPCAM expression [88] express different elements of the BMP pathway. A role for BMP molecules in MaSC regulation was formally demonstrated by functional assay analyses following exposure of different human cell types to soluble BMP2 or BMP4 [76], and further substantiated by the use of TGF/BMP inhibitors allowing the expansion of immature epithelial basal cells [89]. Interestingly, as in the hematopoietic system [90], BMP2 and BMP4 molecules have distinct functional effects on MaSC regulation despite their strong homology. Indeed, while BMP4 modulates the compartment of MaSC and myoepithelial progenitors, BMP2 allows the commitment and proliferation of luminal progenitors [76]. However, the molecular mechanism by which BMPs interact with estrogen signaling to regulate MaSCs remains to be further deciphered.

2.3.2 BMP and breast cancer

BMP signaling is also a well-known highly complex pathway that orchestrates the development and homeostasis of adult tissues such as the neural system [91]. The importance of BMP signaling alterations in cancer stem cell features has been revealed in glioblastoma, breast cancer, and leukemia [90, 92–95]. The role of BMPs, especially of BMP2 and BMP4, in breast cancer has been largely documented [96, 97]. Alterations of BMP ligand expression and signaling have been reported and shown to be clinically correlated with breast cancer progression [98, 99] and to play a major role in the development of bone metastases [99–101]. Despite the fact that BMP4 transcripts are expressed at various levels in tumor tissues or breast cancer cell lines [102], high levels of BMP4 are found in 25% of the breast cancer tumors displaying a low proliferation index but high recurrence rate [98]. BMP4 has crucial functions in promoting tumor growth arrest, migration and metastasis by mediating cell cycle arrest in G1 [102], chemokine regulation [103], and inhibition of lumen formation [104] for example. However, the biological effects of BMP4 largely depend on cell context, as they were reported to be either proliferative or antiproliferative in mammary epithelial cells according to cellular density and cooperative factors [105, 106]. The microenvironment of human primary luminal breast tumors produces abnormally high amounts of soluble BMP2 compared to healthy tissue, while higher BMPR1B levels were detected in tumor cells [76, 107]. Chronic exposure to high BMP2 concentrations was demonstrated to initiate MaSC transformation toward a luminal tumor phenotype dependent on a BMPR1B-initiated signaling cascade involved in luminal commitment of normal MaSC. This leads to a FOXA1/FOXC1 transcription factor balance switch in favor of FOXA1, simultaneously with an upregulation of GATA3 [76]. However, while an increase in soluble BMP2 in the tumor microenvironment has been shown in luminal ER-positive tumors where it is correlated with a high BMPR1B tumor expression [76], a strong decrease in BMP2 transcripts was found in ER-negative breast tumors [108]. Also, a downmodulation of the BMPR1B (Alk6) in a basal cell line (MDA-MB-231) increased cell growth *in vitro* [109], suggesting an antiproliferative function for BMPR1B in ER-negative tumors. Interestingly, downregulation of BMPR1A (ALK3) in MDA-MB231D (a bone metastatic clone of MDA-MB231) basal ER-negative cells inhibited their migration and bone metastatic properties [110]. Therefore, it is very likely that the BMP2/BMPR1B signal is overactivated in the context of ER-positive tumors, while being repressed in ER-negative tumors.

Some of the first steps of carcinogenesis are an increase in proliferation, evasion of apoptosis, and activation of survival signaling pathways. To achieve this, several tumor suppressor genes, like p53 or BRCA1 for instance, need to be inactivated by different mechanisms including epigenetic changes. Modulation of BMP signaling by epigenetic mechanisms [111], such as methylation of BMP-receptor promoters, has been of particular clinical interest to further stratify glioblastoma patients and propose new therapeutic strategies [92]. While different genetic alterations progressively appear following different oncogenic signals, heredity likely accounts for only 10–30% of breast cancers. Based on epidemiological studies, different factors increasing the risk of breast cancer development have been highlighted. They can be intrinsic, like mutations in BRCA1 or 2, Tp53, ATM, or also PTEN, or extrinsic, like environmental factors or lifestyle [112, 113]. In breast cancers with a genetic origin, the most commonly mutated genes are *BRCA1* and *BRCA2,* associated with an increase in cancer risk. BRCA1 and 2 are two major regulators of double-strand breaks (DSB) DNA repair through homologous recombination (HR) and play a crucial role as tumor suppressor genes. In this context, it is interesting to note that a family member and negative regulator of P53, DNp63 has been reported to mediate activation of BMP signaling in order to govern epithelial cell plasticity, EMT, and tumorigenicity during breast cancer initiation and progression [114, 115]. DNp63 has also been identified as a repressor of BRCA1 expression exclusively in ER-positive breast cancer cells [116]. Moreover, a correlation between the BMP pathway and the P53-ATM signaling has been reported [117]. However, the importance of these different signaling crosstalks in the context of breast cancer, exposure to EDCs, and stem cell transformation need to be investigated.

2.4 BMP, estrogen, and bisphenols

2.4.1 BMP and ER crosstalk

The BMP signaling pathway is a dynamic and complex pathway, leading to the transduction of various signals depending on the nature of the BMP ligand and of the BMPR complex oligomerization induced (for review: [118, 119]). It has been shown that BMPs may interact with their receptors in two different ways [120, 121]: on the one hand, BMPs induce a BMPR complex formation called BISC (BMP-induced signaling complex), and on the other hand, a preformed BMPR complex is present before BMP fixation, known as PFC (preformed complex). These two different modes of BMP signal initiation lead to two different signaling cascades, namely the canonical SMAD-dependent pathway and the noncanonical SMAD-independent pathway [121]. SMAD-phosphorylated proteins then form a complex with SMAD4, leading to its translocation to the nucleus where it acts as a transcription factor on target genes [118, 122]. The SMAD-independent pathway does not simply encompass one signaling pathway but a multitude of downstream cascades, involving p38, Ras/ERK, and PI3K/AKT [123–126]. Interestingly, SMAD1-5-8 phosphorylation is more abundant in undifferentiated murine progenitors and decreases with their differentiation until it is almost fully abrogated in the differentiated cells treated with prolactin [87]. Involvement of the BMPR1A/SMAD1-5-8 pathway in lactogenic differentiation was further confirmed by the lack of expression of a lactogenic differentiation marker (beta-casein) at the RNA and protein levels in BMPR1A knockdown mammary cell lines [87]. These data demonstrate that the BMP pathway constitutes an important regulator of the mammary gland during embryogenesis but most likely also during adulthood. However, the molecular and functional crosstalk between the BMP and estrogen signaling pathways is poorly understood. A first set of experiments describes the repression of BMP signaling by ER inhibition of BMP production through a direct interaction between SMAD1 and ER [127]. Reciprocally, a BMP2 signal was shown to upregulate the expression of ER receptors, including the induction of specific ER isoforms such as ERα36 [128, 129]. Interestingly, crosstalk between BMP4 and estrogen signaling seems to have opposite effects. Indeed, BMP4 inhibits ERα signaling by promoting receptor degradation through the proteosomal pathway, while estrogens repress BMP4 expression [130]. Similarly, estrogen represses BMP4 expression in cardiomyocytes by preventing BMP4-mediated ERβ expression and JNK activity in this system [131]. In addition, in this context, estrogen inhibition of BMP4 is independent of Smad1/5/8 activity [131]. BMP4, upon activation of its canonical pathway, represses CYP17A1 and induces the transcription of CYP19A1, involved in androgen and estrogen synthesis, respectively [132]. In a rat model of pituitary cells, estrogen stimulates the transcriptional activity of BMP4-specific SMADs through an ER-SMAD1 complex shown to stimulate prolactin production, while having no effect on the TGFβ/SMAD pathway [133]. Similarly, the inhibitory effects of estrogen signaling on the BMP pathway appear to be mediated by a direct physical interaction between ER receptors and the SMAD1 BMP signaling element in a luminal breast cancer cell line model (MCF7). The physical interaction between ERα and SMAD1 requires the DNA binding domain of ERα and this complex formation is dependent on BMP2 and estrogen [127]. Moreover, BMP signaling has also been directly identified in thyroid-lineage specification [134, 135] as well as in thyroid carcinoma [136]. Interestingly, thyroid hormone status interferes with estrogen target gene expression in breast cancer samples in menopausal women [137]. These findings highlight the need to further investigate the importance of the BMP pathway in both thyroid and estrogen signaling in a broader context of exposure to EDCs.

More recently, BMP2-mediated luminal transformation of MCF10A was shown to be accompanied by a strong activation of the estrogen signaling pathway despite the absence of ERα66 in those cells [76]. Our understanding of estrogen signaling is hindered by the existence of several isoforms generated by alternative splicing and different promoter usage [138]. Interaction of these isoforms with the BMP signaling elements has not yet being investigated but could be involved in epithelial stem cell response to BMP2. Indeed, the importance of these different ERα isoforms in mammary epithelial SC features and in the context of breast cancer is only just starting to be identified [139, 140]. These isoforms can be expressed in both ERα66-positive and -negative cells and display different subcellular localizations [141, 142]. For example, unlike ERα66, ERα36 is expressed mainly at the plasma membrane and activates estrogen nongenomic signaling by activating the ERK pathway through an interplay with the MKP3 phosphatase [143]. Interestingly, in the context of EDC research, ERα36 displays altered ligand preference and causes distinct effects compared to ERα66. For instance, the tamoxifen drug used as an estrogen antagonist in ERα66 breast cancers behaves as an estrogen agonist for ERα36 [140, 144]. Collectively, these different examples illustrate how BMP signaling through its interaction with estrogen signaling is at the crossroad of a number of fundamental physiological processes. The BMP pathway is therefore directly involved in mammary stem cell regulation and transformation, yet adverse effects of EDCs, like BPA, on the BMP pathway have not been thoroughly investigated (**Figure 1**).

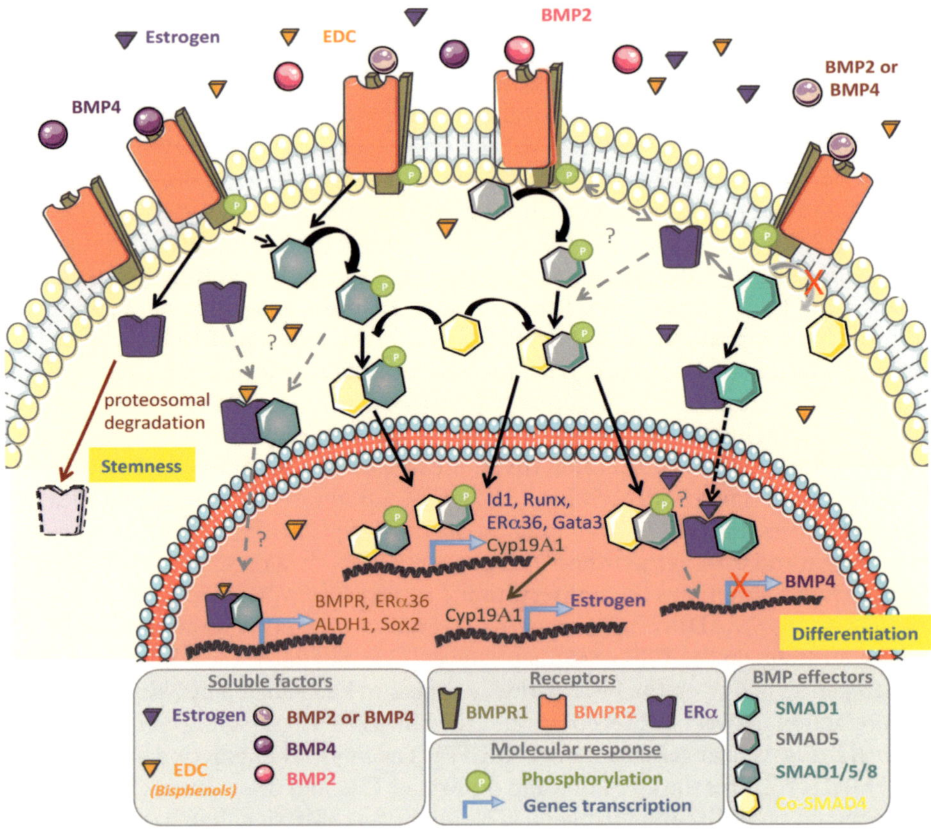

Figure 1.
Illustration of the main findings that show a crosstalk between BMP and estrogen signaling pathways.

2.4.2 BMP and bisphenols

Works from our team and others suggest that bisphenols could act on multiple cell types of the mammary gland, and their effects may converge to provoke major dysregulations of the BMP pathway that could contribute to luminal breast cancer initiation. Indeed, we observed a major impact of BPA on the mammary microenvironment (niche) equilibrium. BPA greatly increases BMP2 production by stromal cells of the human mammary SC microenvironment reaching levels comparable to those measured in luminal breast cancer [76]. Moreover, BPA treatment leads to a decrease in estrogen and BMP15 production in oocytes delaying their maturation [145]. A decrease in BMP2 production through a direct binding of BPA to ERγ was involved in bone loss through a suppression of osteoblast differentiation reverted by inhibition of ERγ [146]. This suggests that the effects and mechanisms of BPA-induced BMP ligand production depend on the estrogen receptor expression profile and are context dependent [147]. However, the molecular mechanism by which BPA induces BMP2 production by stromal cells of the mammary gland BMP2 is not yet known. On the other hand, we have demonstrated that long-term exposure (60 days) to BPA initiates fundamental changes in human mammary stem cells themselves, in particular, by altering major BMP signaling elements such as receptor expression and localization [64]. This results in the "priming" of stem cells to exogenous activating signals of the BMP pathway and sensitizes them to be more sensitive to exogenous soluble BMP ligands. We then demonstrated for the first time that nongenotoxic alterations of both the stem cells and their niche act synergistically to initiate a transforming process mediated by the BMP signaling perturbation leading to the emergence of ER-positive tumors [76]. Interestingly, these previous studies showed that BPA impacts BMP signaling pathway members in both mammary epithelial and stromal cells that do not express ERα66. At the mechanistic level, the pathways used by BPA to induce these effects in cells remain to be deciphered, focusing notably on their reliance on other ERα isoforms or on ER-independent factors.

These questions are of great interest for understanding the effects of both BPA and estrogens since it has been reported that some cell lines respond to an estrogen signal despite their very low levels or complete absence of ER [148]. In response to accumulating evidence in favor of adverse health effects following exposure to BPA, likely mediated by its activation of ERα66, alternative bisphenols have been developed such as BPS and BPF that are considered safer due to their very low binding affinity to ERα [149–151]. However, an increasing number of studies show that these alternative bisphenol molecules are not as innocuous as anticipated, including an impact on obesity, steatosis, and reproduction [20]. In a study previously conducted in our team, assessing the impact of bisphenol on BMP2 production by stromal cells of the mammary gland, we were surprised to observe that BPA and BPS displayed very similar effects [76]. Indeed, both BPA (high affinity binding to estrogen receptors) and its substitute BPS (very weak affinity binding to estrogen receptors) induce BMP2 synthesis in the healthy breast stroma, raising concerns as to whether these bisphenols mediate their transforming effects solely through a classical ER-dependent mechanism. Since then, other studies have shown that BPS, as well as BPF, induces similar if not more potent effects than BPA [20, 152, 153]. Moreover, it was reported that BPA treatment increases aromatase expression and its activity in healthy breast fibroblasts, leading to an increase in estrogen biosynthesis and secretion. The same observations were made after treatment with BPS [154]. These results are of particular interest with regards to the important role of the microenvironment in the different steps of carcinogenesis and in the context of MaSC-driven transformation by BMP signaling. Our work thus indicates that the BMP pathway could be altered by several EDCs such as BPA and its proposed alternatives, both at the level of stem cells and their microenvironment. This suggests that early detection of increased BMP2 levels in the mammary microenvironment may constitute a reliable marker of early transformation process and could be a valuable indicator of exposure to EDCs such as bisphenols. In addition, the interplay between BMP and estrogen pathways both at the molecular and functional levels prompt us to further decipher the mechanisms underlying bisphenol- and BMP-induced transformation in mammary epithelial stem cells.

3. Conclusions

Different signaling pathways often engage in complex interactions synergistically mediating an appropriate cellular response. Estrogen signaling is no exception and it is likely involved in a crosstalk with the BMP pathway at multiple levels in the mammary gland. BMPs are secreted proteins active in a very large number of organs and tissues during development, adulthood, and pathogenesis [155]. Previous work suggested a close interaction between ER-mediated estrogen signaling and the BMP pathway in different cell types of the mammary gland. In a model of mammary epithelial stem cells, E2 or known EDCs like BPA or BPS were able to potentiate SMAD activation by BMP2 [64]. This was possibly due to a physical interaction between ERα isoforms and SMAD factors, such as that reported for ERα or ERβ, and could be associated with an increased risk of cell transformation by long-term exposure to BMP2.

Deciphering the dysregulations of the BMP signaling pathway has been remarkably useful in identifying its importance in cancer stem cell phenotypes in the neural system [92, 93]. The role of alterations of BMP signaling to sustain cancer stem cell features has been extended by us and others in breast cancer and leukemia [90, 94, 95]. We showed that chronic exposure to high concentrations of BMP2 drives the transformation of mammary stem cells toward the luminal tumor subtype [76] through binding to its BMPR1B receptor. However, downstream mechanisms and crosstalks with estrogen signaling in those mammary stem cells remained to be understood. This is especially important in the context of several studies that demonstrated the involvement of BPA in the proliferation of either ER-positive or -negative cancer cells. In addition, BPA can trigger proliferation via nonclassical estrogen receptors, including the estrogen-related receptor gamma (ERRγ) [156, 157]. We also demonstrated that long-term exposure of human mammary stem cells (ER-negative in terms of ERα-66 expression) to pollutants such as BPA initiates fundamental changes in stem cells by altering major BMP signaling components [64], thus "priming" stem cells to exogenous BMP activation. Complementary to this effect on epithelial stem cells, we revealed an impact of BPA on the tumor microenvironment through the induction of the synthesis of high levels of BMP2 by normal fibroblasts and stromal cells reaching levels similar to those measured in breast tumors [76].

Resistance and relapse can be due to tumor adaptation or evolution. Indeed, therapies elicit a selective pressure on cells, which in turn develop resistance, notably by acquiring mutations. Resistance to tamoxifen of ER-positive tumors can be caused by a loss of ER [158], its mutation, or posttranslational modification [159] among others. It was shown that BPA is involved in chemoresistance [160] and notably in resistance to tamoxifen in ER-positive tumor cell lines [161] by decreasing tamoxifen-induced apoptosis and increasing gene expression of ERRα, which contributes to resistance to tamoxifen [162] and cell proliferation [157]. Another study demonstrated that an ERα variant could be induced by BMP2 [128] and may be involved in resistance to tamoxifen [163]. The addiction of cancer cells toward BMP signaling and the crosstalk with estrogen signaling is currently under consideration as a new therapeutic avenue for ER-positive breast cancer patients [164]. At the clinical level, targeting estrogen signaling has been decisive in improving the outcome of ER-positive breast cancer patients. At the era of immunotherapy, the analysis of the impact of bisphenols on the immune system and on tumor surveillance is crucial. This will need to be pursued to improve our understanding and implementation of antiestrogen therapies in the context of their combination with new immune treatments [165]. Overall, these data indicate that disruption of BMP signaling affects both the stem cells and their niche at different stages of the disease, which could be instrumental in the management of breast cancer.

Several studies demonstrated that BPS promotes breast cancer cell proliferation, notably through an ER-cyclin D1-CDK4/6-pRb-dependent pathway, exclusively in ER-positive breast cancer cells [38, 39, 166]. Moreover, it has also been demonstrated that BPF has the same proliferative action as BPA, BPS, or estrogen treatments on transformed ER-positive cells. Similar to BPS, this proliferative effect relies on cyclin D and E expression through ER-dependent pathways [39]. BPS, as shown for BPA, can also induce epigenetic and transcriptional changes in breast cancer cells, resulting in an increase in the expression of genes implicated in proliferation, cellular attachment as well as adhesion and migration [167]. Lastly, the bioavailability of BPS substitutes might be higher than for BPA. A recent study conducted in pigs, an ideal model for mimicking the human digestive tract, demonstrated the lower plasma clearance of BPS (3.5 lower) compared to BPA and an increased oral systemic exposure exceeding 250-fold [168]. These observations draw our attention and raise concerns about replacing BPA by BPS, as this may result in an increased internal exposure to EDCs.

To conclude, BMP signaling plays a major role in the regulation of SCs and of their microenvironment (niche), in both normal and tumor contexts. Multiple abnormalities of BMP signaling have been observed in cancer, but until recently studies had mostly focused on its role in advanced disease. However, due to the number of studies describing the importance of BMP signaling throughout breast cancer development (from initiation, progression, metastasis up to resistance), we suggest that early detection of BMP signaling alterations, such as increased levels of BMP2 and/or of BMP receptors, may constitute a reliable marker of exposure to BPA. This suggests that further investigations into alterations of the BMP pathway in the context of exposure to bisphenols should improve our understanding of associated side effects.

Acknowledgements

The authors thank the following funding bodies for their support of the team's work mentioned in this review: the Association pour la Recherche contre le Cancer, La Ligue contre le Cancer, the Déchaine ton cœur association, the Région Rhône-Alpes and the Institut National du Cancer.

Conflict of interest

The authors declare no conflict of interest.

Notes/thanks/other declarations

The author thanks Brigitte Manship for English proofreading and critical reading.

Author details

Boris Guyot and Veronique Maguer-Satta*
Université Claude Bernard Lyon 1, Cancer Research Center of Lyon-CRCL, CNRS UMR5286, Inserm U1052, Lyon Cedex, France

*Address all correspondence to: veronique.maguer-satta@lyon.unicancer.fr

References

[1] Pourteimoor V, Mohammadi-Yeganeh S, Paryan M. Breast cancer classification and prognostication through diverse systems along with recent emerging findings in this respect; the dawn of new perspectives in the clinical applications. Tumour Biology. 2016;**37**(11):14479-14499

[2] Goldhirsch A, Winer EP, Coates AS, Gelber RD, Piccart-Gebhart M, Thurlimann B, et al. Personalizing the treatment of women with early breast cancer: Highlights of the St Gallen International Expert Consensus on the Primary Therapy of Early Breast Cancer 2013. Annals of Oncology. 2013;**24**(9):2206-2223

[3] Sorlie T, Perou CM, Tibshirani R, Aas T, Geisler S, Johnsen H, et al. Gene expression patterns of breast carcinomas distinguish tumor subclasses with clinical implications. Proceedings of the National Academy of Sciences of the United States of America. 2001;**98**(19):10869-10874

[4] Lumachi F, Santeufemia DA, Basso SM. Current medical treatment of estrogen receptor-positive breast cancer. World Journal of Biological Chemistry. 2015;**6**(3):231-239

[5] Momenimovahed Z, Salehiniya H. Epidemiological characteristics of and risk factors for breast cancer in the world. Breast Cancer (Dove Medical Press). 2019;**11**:151-164

[6] WHO IPoCS. Global assessment of the state-of-the-science of endocrine disruptors. 2002

[7] WHO/UNEP. State of the science of endocrine disrupting chemicals—2012. 2012

[8] Goodson WH 3rd, Lowe L, Carpenter DO, Gilbertson M, Manaf Ali A, Lopez de Cerain Salsamendi A, et al. Assessing the carcinogenic potential of low-dose exposures to chemical mixtures in the environment: The challenge ahead. Carcinogenesis. 2015;**36**(Suppl 1):S254-S296

[9] Kabir ER, Rahman MS, Rahman I. A review on endocrine disruptors and their possible impacts on human health. Environmental Toxicology and Pharmacology. 2015;**40**(1):241-258

[10] Gore AC, Chappell VA, Fenton SE, Flaws JA, Nadal A, Prins GS, et al. EDC-2: The endocrine society's second scientific statement on endocrine-disrupting chemicals. Endocrine Reviews. 2015;**36**(6):E1-E150

[11] Zoeller RT, Brown TR, Doan LL, Gore AC, Skakkebaek NE, Soto AM, et al. Endocrine-disrupting chemicals and public health protection: A statement of principles from the Endocrine Society. Endocrinology. 2012;**153**(9):4097-4110

[12] Li Y, Perera L, Coons LA, Burns KA, Tyler Ramsey J, Pelch KE, et al. Differential in vitro biological action, coregulator interactions, and molecular dynamic analysis of Bisphenol A (BPA), BPAF, and BPS ligand-ERalpha complexes. Environmental Health Perspectives. 2018;**126**(1):017012

[13] Routledge EJ, White R, Parker MG, Sumpter JP. Differential effects of xenoestrogens on coactivator recruitment by estrogen receptor (ER) alpha and ERbeta. The Journal of Biological Chemistry. 2000;**275**(46):35986-35993

[14] Rochester JR. Bisphenol A and human health: A review of the literature. Reproductive Toxicology. 2013;**42**:132-155

[15] Alonso-Magdalena P, Ropero AB, Soriano S, Garcia-Arevalo M, Ripoll C, Fuentes E, et al. Bisphenol-A acts as a potent estrogen via non-classical estrogen triggered pathways. Molecular and Cellular Endocrinology. 2012;**355**(2):201-207

[16] Hammes SR, Levin ER. Extranuclear steroid receptors: Nature and actions. Endocrine Reviews. 2007;**28**(7):726-741

[17] MacKay H, Abizaid A. A plurality of molecular targets: The receptor ecosystem for bisphenol-A (BPA). Hormones and Behavior. 2018;**101**:59-67

[18] Wang T, Liu B, Guan Y, Gong M, Zhang W, Pan J, et al. Melatonin inhibits the proliferation of breast cancer cells induced by bisphenol A via targeting estrogen receptor-related pathways. Thoracic Cancer. 2018;**9**(3):368-375

[19] Murata M, Kang JH. Bisphenol A (BPA) and cell signaling pathways. Biotechnology Advances. 2018;**36**(1):311-327

[20] Siracusa JS, Yin L, Measel E, Liang S, Yu X. Effects of bisphenol A and its analogs on reproductive health: A mini review. Reproductive Toxicology. 2018;**79**:96-123

[21] Urriola-Munoz P, Li X, Maretzky T, McIlwain DR, Mak TW, Reyes JG, et al. The xenoestrogens biphenol-A and nonylphenol differentially regulate metalloprotease-mediated shedding of EGFR ligands. Journal of Cellular Physiology. 2018;**233**(3):2247-2256

[22] Watson CS, Bulayeva NN, Wozniak AL, Alyea RA. Xenoestrogens are potent activators of nongenomic estrogenic responses. Steroids. 2007;**72**(2):124-134

[23] Holmes D. Breast cancer: Increased risk with concurrent dietary and EDC exposures. Nature Reviews. Endocrinology. 2017;**13**(7):378

[24] Hussain I, Bhan A, Ansari KI, Deb P, Bobzean SA, Perrotti LI, et al. Bisphenol-A induces expression of HOXC6, an estrogen-regulated homeobox-containing gene associated with breast cancer. Biochimica et Biophysica Acta. 2015;**1849**(6):697-708

[25] Hafezi SA, Abdel-Rahman WM. The endocrine disruptor Bisphenol A (BPA) exerts a wide range of effects in carcinogenesis and response to therapy. Current Molecular Pharmacology. 2019;**12**(3):230-238;

[26] Sprague BL, Trentham-Dietz A, Hedman CJ, Wang J, Hemming JD, Hampton JM, et al. Circulating serum xenoestrogens and mammographic breast density. Breast Cancer Research. 2013;**15**(3):R45

[27] Ayyanan A, Laribi O, Schuepbach-Mallepell S, Schrick C, Gutierrez M, Tanos T, et al. Perinatal exposure to bisphenol a increases adult mammary gland progesterone response and cell number. Molecular Endocrinology. 2011;**25**(11):1915-1923

[28] Gao H, Yang BJ, Li N, Feng LM, Shi XY, Zhao WH, et al. Bisphenol A and hormone-associated cancers: Current progress and perspectives. Medicine (Baltimore). 2015;**94**(1):e211

[29] Fernandez SV, Russo J. Estrogen and xenoestrogens in breast cancer. Toxicologic Pathology. 2010;**38**(1):110-122

[30] Dairkee SH, Seok J, Champion S, Sayeed A, Mindrinos M, Xiao W, et al. Bisphenol A induces a profile of tumor aggressiveness in high-risk cells from breast cancer patients. Cancer Research. 2008;**68**(7):2076-2080

[31] Seyfried TN, Huysentruyt LC. On the origin of cancer metastasis. Critical Reviews in Oncogenesis. 2013;**18**(1-2):43-73

[32] Weigelt B, Peterse JL, Van't Veer LJ. Breast cancer metastasis: Markers and models. Nature Reviews. Cancer. 2005;**5**(8):591-602

[33] Gupta GP, Massague J. Cancer metastasis: Building a framework. Cell. 2006;**127**(4):679-695

[34] Jin X, Mu P. Targeting breast cancer metastasis. Breast Cancer (Auckl.). 2015;**9**(Suppl 1):23-34

[35] Rangel R, Guzman-Rojas L, Kodama T, Kodama M, Newberg JY, Copeland NG, et al. Identification of new tumor suppressor genes in triple-negative breast cancer. Cancer Research. 2017;**77**(15): 4089-4101

[36] Zhang XL, Wang HS, Liu N, Ge LC. Bisphenol A stimulates the epithelial mesenchymal transition of estrogen negative breast cancer cells via FOXA1 signals. Archives of Biochemistry and Biophysics. 2015;**585**:10-16

[37] Castillo Sanchez R, Gomez R, Perez Salazar E. Bisphenol A induces migration through a GPER-, FAK-, Src-, and ERK2-dependent pathway in MDA-MB-231 breast cancer cells. Chemical Research in Toxicology. 2016;**29**(3):285-295

[38] Deng Q, Jiang G, Wu Y, Li J, Liang W, Chen L, et al. GPER/hippo-YAP signal is involved in Bisphenol S induced migration of triple negative breast cancer (TNBC) cells. Journal of Hazardous Materials. 2018;**355**:1-9

[39] Kim JY, Choi HG, Lee HM, Lee GA, Hwang KA, Choi KC. Effects of bisphenol compounds on the growth and epithelial mesenchymal transition of MCF-7 CV human breast cancer cells. Journal of Biomedical Research. 2017;**31**(4):358-369

[40] Shafei A, Matbouly M, Mostafa E, Al Sannat S, Abdelrahman M, Lewis B, et al. Stop eating plastic, molecular signaling of bisphenol A in breast cancer. Environmental Science and Pollution Research International. 2018;**25**(24):23624-23630

[41] Morgan M, Deoraj A, Felty Q, Roy D. Environmental estrogen-like endocrine disrupting chemicals and breast cancer. Molecular and Cellular Endocrinology. 2017;**457**:89-102

[42] Shafei A, Ramzy MM, Hegazy AI, Husseny AK, El-Hadary UG, Taha MM, et al. The molecular mechanisms of action of the endocrine disrupting chemical bisphenol A in the development of cancer. Gene. 2018;**647**:235-243

[43] Silberstein GB, Van Horn K, Shyamala G, Daniel CW. Essential role of endogenous estrogen in directly stimulating mammary growth demonstrated by implants containing pure antiestrogens. Endocrinology. 1994;**134**(1):84-90

[44] Feng Y, Manka D, Wagner KU, Khan SA. Estrogen receptor-alpha expression in the mammary epithelium is required for ductal and alveolar morphogenesis in mice. Proceedings of the National Academy of Sciences of the United States of America. 2007;**104**(37):14718-14723

[45] Daniel CW, Silberstein GB, Strickland P. Direct action of 17 beta-estradiol on mouse mammary ducts analyzed by sustained release implants and steroid autoradiography. Cancer Research. 1987;**47**(22):6052-6057

[46] Lydon JP, Sivaraman L, Conneely OM. A reappraisal of progesterone action in the mammary gland. Journal of Mammary Gland Biology and Neoplasia. 2000;**5**(3):325-338

[47] Shyamala G. Progesterone signaling and mammary gland morphogenesis.

Journal of Mammary Gland Biology and Neoplasia. 1999;**4**(1):89-104

[48] Stingl J, Eirew P, Ricketson I, Shackleton M, Vaillant F, Choi D, et al. Purification and unique properties of mammary epithelial stem cells. Nature. 2006;**439**(7079):993-997

[49] Shackleton M, Vaillant F, Simpson KJ, Stingl J, Smyth GK, Asselin-Labat ML, et al. Generation of a functional mammary gland from a single stem cell. Nature. 2006;**439**(7072):84-88

[50] Inman JL, Robertson C, Mott JD, Bissell MJ. Mammary gland development: Cell fate specification, stem cells and the microenvironment. Development. 2015;**142**(6):1028-1042

[51] Lloyd-Lewis B, Harris OB, Watson CJ, Davis FM. Mammary stem cells: Premise, properties, and perspectives. Trends in Cell Biology. 2017;**27**(8):556-567

[52] Asselin-Labat ML, Vaillant F, Sheridan JM, Pal B, Wu D, Simpson ER, et al. Control of mammary stem cell function by steroid hormone signalling. Nature. 2010;**465**(7299):798-802

[53] Brisken C. Hormonal control of alveolar development and its implications for breast carcinogenesis. Journal of Mammary Gland Biology and Neoplasia. 2002;**7**(1):39-48

[54] Humphreys RC, Lydon JP, O'Malley BW, Rosen JM. Use of PRKO mice to study the role of progesterone in mammary gland development. Journal of Mammary Gland Biology and Neoplasia. 1997;**2**(4):343-354

[55] Mallepell S, Krust A, Chambon P, Brisken C. Paracrine signaling through the epithelial estrogen receptor alpha is required for proliferation and morphogenesis in the mammary gland. Proceedings of the National Academy of Sciences of the United States of America. 2006;**103**(7):2196-2201

[56] Stingl J. Estrogen and progesterone in normal mammary gland development and in cancer. Hormones and Cancer. 2011;**2**(2):85-90

[57] Ciarloni L, Mallepell S, Brisken C. Amphiregulin is an essential mediator of estrogen receptor alpha function in mammary gland development. Proceedings of the National Academy of Sciences of the United States of America. 2007;**104**(13):5455-5460

[58] LaMarca HL, Rosen JM. Estrogen regulation of mammary gland development and breast cancer: Amphiregulin takes center stage. Breast Cancer Research. 2007;**9**(4):304

[59] Sternlicht MD, Sunnarborg SW, Kouros-Mehr H, Yu Y, Lee DC, Werb Z. Mammary ductal morphogenesis requires paracrine activation of stromal EGFR via ADAM17-dependent shedding of epithelial amphiregulin. Development. 2005;**132**(17):3923-3933

[60] Villadsen R, Fridriksdottir AJ, Ronnov-Jessen L, Gudjonsson T, Rank F, LaBarge MA, et al. Evidence for a stem cell hierarchy in the adult human breast. Journal of Cell Biology. 2007;**177**(1):87-101

[61] Booth BW, Smith GH. ERalpha and PR are expressed in label-retaining mammary epithelial cells that divide asymmetrically and retain their template DNA strands. Breast Cancer Research. 2006;**8**(4):R49

[62] Booth BW, Boulanger CA, Anderson LH, Jimenez-Rojo L, Brisken C, Smith GH. Amphiregulin mediates self-renewal in an immortal mammary epithelial cell line with stem cell characteristics. Experimental Cell Research. 2010;**316**(3):422-432

[63] Russo J, Snider K, Pereira JS, Russo IH. Estrogen induced breast cancer is the result in the disruption of the asymmetric cell division of the stem cell. Hormone Molecular Biology and Clinical Investigation. 2010;**1**(2):53-65

[64] Clement F, Xu X, Donini CF, Clement A, Omarjee S, Delay E, et al. Long-term exposure to bisphenol A or benzo(a)pyrene alters the fate of human mammary epithelial stem cells in response to BMP2 and BMP4, by pre-activating BMP signaling. Cell Death and Differentiation. 2017;**24**(1):155-166

[65] Kopras E, Potluri V, Bermudez ML, Williams K, Belcher S, Kasper S. Actions of endocrine-disrupting chemicals on stem/progenitor cells during development and disease. Endocrine-Related Cancer. 2014;**21**(2):T1-T12

[66] Bateman ME, Strong AL, McLachlan JA, Burow ME, Bunnell BA. The effects of endocrine disruptors on adipogenesis and osteogenesis in mesenchymal stem cells: A review. Frontiers in Endocrinology. 2016;**7**:171

[67] Alonso-Magdalena P, Rivera FJ, Guerrero-Bosagna C. Bisphenol-A and metabolic diseases: Epigenetic, developmental and transgenerational basis. Environmental Epigenetics. 2016;**2**(3):dvw022

[68] Landero-Huerta DA, Vigueras-Villasenor RM, Yokoyama-Rebollar E, Arechaga-OcampoE,Rojas-CastanedaJC, Jimenez-Trejo F, et al. Epigenetic and risk factors of testicular germ cell tumors: A brief review. Frontiers in Bioscience (Landmark Edition). 2017;**22**:1073-1098

[69] Moral R, Wang R, Russo IH, Lamartiniere CA, Pereira J, Russo J. Effect of prenatal exposure to the endocrine disruptor bisphenol A on mammary gland morphology and gene expression signature. The Journal of Endocrinology. 2008;**196**(1):101-112

[70] Vandenberg LN, Maffini MV, Wadia PR, Sonnenschein C, Rubin BS, Soto AM. Exposure to environmentally relevant doses of the xenoestrogen bisphenol-A alters development of the fetal mouse mammary gland. Endocrinology. 2007;**148**(1):116-127

[71] Wadia PR, Cabaton NJ, Borrero MD, Rubin BS, Sonnenschein C, Shioda T, et al. Low-dose BPA exposure alters the mesenchymal and epithelial transcriptomes of the mouse fetal mammary gland. PLoS One. 2013;**8**(5):e63902

[72] Wang D, Gao H, Bandyopadhyay A, Wu A, Yeh IT, Chen Y, et al. Pubertal bisphenol A exposure alters murine mammary stem cell function leading to early neoplasia in regenerated glands. Cancer Prevention Research (Philadelphia, Pa.). 2014;**7**(4):445-455

[73] Qin XY, Fukuda T, Yang L, Zaha H, Akanuma H, Zeng Q, et al. Effects of bisphenol A exposure on the proliferation and senescence of normal human mammary epithelial cells. Cancer Biology & Therapy. 2012;**13**(5):296-306

[74] Fernandez SV, Huang Y, Snider KE, Zhou Y, Pogash TJ, Russo J. Expression and DNA methylation changes in human breast epithelial cells after bisphenol A exposure. International Journal of Oncology. 2012;**41**(1):369-377

[75] Lillo MA, Nichols C, Seagroves TN, Miranda-Carboni GA, Krum SA. Bisphenol A induces Sox2 in ER(+) breast cancer stem-like cells. Hormones and Cancer. 2017;**8**(2):90-99

[76] Chapellier M, Bachelard-Cascales E, Schmidt X, Clement F, Treilleux I, Delay E, et al. Disequilibrium of BMP2 levels in the breast stem cell niche

launches epithelial transformation by overamplifying BMPR1B cell response. Stem Cell Reports. 2015;**4**(2):239-254

[77] Wang RN, Green J, Wang Z, Deng Y, Qiao M, Peabody M, et al. Bone morphogenetic protein (BMP) signaling in development and human diseases. Genes & Diseases. 2014;**1**(1):87-105

[78] Huang RL, Sun Y, Ho CK, Liu K, Tang QQ, Xie Y, et al. IL-6 potentiates BMP-2-induced osteogenesis and adipogenesis via two different BMPR1A-mediated pathways. Cell Death & Disease. 2018;**9**(2):144

[79] Zhang X, Guo J, Zhou Y, Wu G. The roles of bone morphogenetic proteins and their signaling in the osteogenesis of adipose-derived stem cells. Tissue Engineering. Part B, Reviews. 2014;**20**(1):84-92

[80] Gustafson B, Hammarstedt A, Hedjazifar S, Hoffmann JM, Svensson PA, Grimsby J, et al. BMP4 and BMP antagonists regulate human white and beige adipogenesis. Diabetes. 2015;**64**(5):1670-1681

[81] Ribeiro S, Lopes LR, Paula Costa G, Figueiredo VP, Shrestha D, Batista AP, et al. CXCL-16, IL-17, and bone morphogenetic protein 2 (BMP-2) are associated with overweight and obesity conditions in middle-aged and elderly women. Immunity & Ageing. 2017;**14**:6

[82] Zamani N, Brown CW. Emerging roles for the transforming growth factor-{beta} superfamily in regulating adiposity and energy expenditure. Endocrine Reviews. 2011;**32**(3):387-403

[83] Cho KW, Kim JY, Song SJ, Farrell E, Eblaghie MC, Kim HJ, et al. Molecular interactions between Tbx3 and Bmp4 and a model for dorsoventral positioning of mammary gland development. Proceedings of the National Academy of Sciences of the United States of America. 2006;**103**(45):16788-16793

[84] Hens JR, Dann P, Zhang JP, Harris S, Robinson GW, Wysolmerski J. BMP4 and PTHrP interact to stimulate ductal outgrowth during embryonic mammary development and to inhibit hair follicle induction. Development. 2007;**134**(6):1221-1230

[85] Fleming JM, Ginsburg E, Goldhar AS, Plant J, Vonderhaar BK. Progesterone receptor activates Msx2 expression by downregulating TNAP/Akp2 and activating the Bmp pathway in EpH4 mouse mammary epithelial cells. PLoS One. 2012;**7**(3):e34058

[86] Forsman CL, Ng BC, Heinze RK, Kuo C, Sergi C, Gopalakrishnan R, et al. BMP-binding protein twisted gastrulation is required in mammary gland epithelium for normal ductal elongation and myoepithelial compartmentalization. Developmental Biology. 2013;**373**(1):95-106

[87] Perotti C, Karayazi O, Moffat S, Shemanko CS. The bone morphogenetic protein receptor-1A pathway is required for lactogenic differentiation of mammary epithelial cells in vitro. In Vitro Cellular & Developmental Biology—Animal. 2012;**48**(6):377-384

[88] Bachelard-Cascales E, Chapellier M, Delay E, Pochon G, Voeltzel T, Puisieux A, et al. The CD10 enzyme is a key player to identify and regulate human mammary stem cells. Stem Cells. 2010;**28**(6):1081-1088

[89] Mou H, Vinarsky V, Tata PR, Brazauskas K, Choi SH, Crooke AK, et al. Dual SMAD signaling inhibition enables long-term expansion of diverse epithelial basal cells. Cell Stem Cell. 2016;**19**(2):217-231

[90] Zylbersztejn F, Flores-Violante M, Voeltzel T, Nicolini FE, Lefort S,

Maguer-Satta V. The BMP pathway: A unique tool to decode the origin and progression of leukemia. Experimental Hematology. 2018;**61**:36-44

[91] Bier E, De Robertis EM. Embryo development. BMP gradients: A paradigm for morphogen-mediated developmental patterning. Science. 2015;**348**(6242):aaa5838

[92] Lee J, Son MJ, Woolard K, Donin NM, Li A, Cheng CH, et al. Epigenetic-mediated dysfunction of the bone morphogenetic protein pathway inhibits differentiation of glioblastoma-initiating cells. Cancer Cell. 2008;**13**(1):69-80

[93] Piccirillo SG, Reynolds BA, Zanetti N, Lamorte G, Binda E, Broggi G, et al. Bone morphogenetic proteins inhibit the tumorigenic potential of human brain tumour-initiating cells. Nature. 2006;**444**(7120):761-765

[94] Jung N, Maguer-Satta V, Guyot B. Early steps of mammary stem cells transformation by exogenous signals, effects of the bisphenols endocrine disruptors. Cancers. 2019;**11**(9): 1351-1368

[95] Chapellier M, Maguer-Satta V. BMP2, a key to uncover luminal breast cancer origin linked to pollutant effects on epithelial stem cells niche. Molecular & Cellular Oncology. 2016;**3**(3):e1026527

[96] Alarmo EL, Kallioniemi A. Bone morphogenetic proteins in breast cancer: Dual role in tumourigenesis? Endocrine-Related Cancer. 2010;**17**(2):R123-RR39

[97] Thawani JP, Wang AC, Than KD, Lin CY, La Marca F, Park P. Bone morphogenetic proteins and cancer: Review of the literature. Neurosurgery. 2010;**66**(2):233-246

[98] Alarmo EL, Huhtala H, Korhonen T, Pylkkanen L, Holli K, Kuukasjarvi T, et al. Bone morphogenetic protein 4 expression in multiple normal and tumor tissues reveals its importance beyond development. Modern Pathology: An Official Journal of the United States and Canadian Academy of Pathology, Inc. 2013;**26**(1):10-21

[99] Zabkiewicz C, Resaul J, Hargest R, Jiang WG, Ye L. Bone morphogenetic proteins, breast cancer, and bone metastases: Striking the right balance. Endocrine-Related Cancer. 2017;**24**(10):R349-RR66

[100] Ye L, Jiang WG. Bone morphogenetic proteins in tumour associated angiogenesis and implication in cancer therapies. Cancer Letters. 2016;**380**(2):586-597

[101] Bellanger A, Donini CF, Vendrell JA, Lavaud J, Machuca-Gayet I, Ruel M, et al. The critical role of the ZNF217 oncogene in promoting breast cancer metastasis to the bone. The Journal of Pathology. 2017;**242**(1):73-89

[102] Ketolainen JM, Alarmo EL, Tuominen VJ, Kallioniemi A. Parallel inhibition of cell growth and induction of cell migration and invasion in breast cancer cells by bone morphogenetic protein 4. Breast Cancer Research and Treatment. 2010;**124**(2):377-386

[103] Owens P, Pickup MW, Novitskiy SV, Chytil A, Gorska AE, Aakre ME, et al. Disruption of bone morphogenetic protein receptor 2 (BMPR2) in mammary tumors promotes metastases through cell autonomous and paracrine mediators. Proceedings of the National Academy of Sciences of the United States of America. 2012;**109**(8):2814-2819

[104] Montesano R. Bone morphogenetic protein-4 abrogates lumen formation by mammary epithelial cells and promotes invasive growth. Biochemical and Biophysical Research Communications. 2007;**353**(3):817-822

[105] Masuda H, Otsuka F, Matsumoto Y, Takano M, Miyoshi T, Inagaki K, et al. Functional interaction of fibroblast growth factor-8, bone morphogenetic protein and estrogen receptor in breast cancer cell proliferation. Molecular and Cellular Endocrinology. 2011;**343**(1-2):7-17

[106] Montesano R, Sarkozi R, Schramek H. Bone morphogenetic protein-4 strongly potentiates growth factor-induced proliferation of mammary epithelial cells. Biochemical and Biophysical Research Communications. 2008;**374**(1):164-168

[107] Helms MW, Packeisen J, August C, Schittek B, Boecker W, Brandt BH, et al. First evidence supporting a potential role for the BMP/SMAD pathway in the progression of oestrogen receptor-positive breast cancer. Journal of Pathology. 2005;**206**(3):366-376

[108] Arnold SF, Tims E, McGrath BE. Identification of bone morphogenetic proteins and their receptors in human breast cancer cell lines: Importance of BMP2. Cytokine. 1999;**11**(12):1031-1037

[109] Bokobza SM, Ye L, Kynaston HE, Mansel RE, Jiang WG. Reduced expression of BMPR-IB correlates with poor prognosis and increased proliferation of breast cancer cells. Cancer Genomics & Proteomics. 2009;**6**(2):101-108

[110] Katsuno Y, Hanyu A, Kanda H, Ishikawa Y, Akiyama F, Iwase T, et al. Bone morphogenetic protein signaling enhances invasion and bone metastasis of breast cancer cells through Smad pathway. Oncogene. 2008;**27**(49):6322-6333

[111] Zhang M, Wang Q, Yuan W, Yang S, Wang X, Yan JD, et al. Epigenetic regulation of bone morphogenetic protein-6 gene expression in breast cancer cells. The Journal of Steroid Biochemistry and Molecular Biology. 2007;**105**(1-5):91-97

[112] Lal A, Ramazzotti D, Weng Z, Liu K, Ford JM, Sidow A. Comprehensive genomic characterization of breast tumors with BRCA1 and BRCA2 mutations. BMC Medical Genomics. 2019;**12**(1):84

[113] Lima ZS, Ghadamzadeh M, Arashloo FT, Amjad G, Ebadi MR, Younesi L. Recent advances of therapeutic targets based on the molecular signature in breast cancer: Genetic mutations and implications for current treatment paradigms. Journal of Hematology & Oncology. 2019;**12**(1):38

[114] Balboni AL, Hutchinson JA, DeCastro AJ, Cherukuri P, Liby K, Sporn MB, et al. DeltaNp63alpha-mediated activation of bone morphogenetic protein signaling governs stem cell activity and plasticity in normal and malignant mammary epithelial cells. Cancer Research. 2013;**73**(2):1020-1030

[115] DeCastro AJ, Cherukuri P, Balboni A, DiRenzo J. DeltaNP63alpha transcriptionally activates chemokine receptor 4 (CXCR4) expression to regulate breast cancer stem cell activity and chemotaxis. Molecular Cancer Therapeutics. 2015;**14**(1):225-235

[116] Amin R, Morita-Fujimura Y, Tawarayama H, Semba K, Chiba N, Fukumoto M, et al. DeltaNp63alpha induces quiescence and downregulates the BRCA1 pathway in estrogen receptor-positive luminal breast cancer cell line MCF7 but not in other breast cancer cell lines. Molecular Oncology. 2016;**10**(4):575-593

[117] Chau JF, Jia D, Wang Z, Liu Z, Hu Y, Zhang X, et al. A crucial role for bone morphogenetic protein-Smad1 signalling in the DNA damage response. Nature Communications. 2012;**3**:836

[118] Miyazono K, Maeda S, Imamura T. BMP receptor signaling: Transcriptional targets, regulation of signals, and signaling cross-talk. Cytokine & Growth Factor Reviews. 2005;**16**(3):251-263

[119] Yadin D, Knaus P, Mueller TD. Structural insights into BMP receptors: Specificity, activation and inhibition. Cytokine & Growth Factor Reviews. 2016;**27**:13-34

[120] Nohe A, Hassel S, Ehrlich M, Neubauer F, Sebald W, Henis YI, et al. The mode of bone morphogenetic protein (BMP) receptor oligomerization determines different BMP-2 signaling pathways. The Journal of Biological Chemistry. 2002;**277**(7):5330-5338

[121] Hassel S, Schmitt S, Hartung A, Roth M, Nohe A, Petersen N, et al. Initiation of Smad-dependent and Smad-independent signaling via distinct BMP-receptor complexes. The Journal of Bone and Joint Surgery. American Volume. 2003;**85-A**(Suppl 3):44-51

[122] Miyazono K, Kamiya Y, Morikawa M. Bone morphogenetic protein receptors and signal transduction. Journal of Biochemistry. 2010;**147**(1):35-51

[123] Gamell C, Osses N, Bartrons R, Ruckle T, Camps M, Rosa JL, et al. BMP2 induction of actin cytoskeleton reorganization and cell migration requires PI3-kinase and Cdc42 activity. Journal of Cell Science. 2008;**121**(Pt 23):3960-3970

[124] Guicheux J, Lemonnier J, Ghayor C, Suzuki A, Palmer G, Caverzasio J. Activation of p38 mitogen-activated protein kinase and c-Jun-NH2-terminal kinase by BMP-2 and their implication in the stimulation of osteoblastic cell differentiation. Journal of Bone and Mineral Research. 2003;**18**(11):2060-2068

[125] Hay E, Lemonnier J, Fromigue O, Marie PJ. Bone morphogenetic protein-2 promotes osteoblast apoptosis through a Smad-independent, protein kinase C-dependent signaling pathway. The Journal of Biological Chemistry. 2001;**276**(31):29028-29036

[126] Vinals F, Lopez-Rovira T, Rosa JL, Ventura F. Inhibition of PI3K/p70 S6K and p38 MAPK cascades increases osteoblastic differentiation induced by BMP-2. FEBS Letters. 2002;**510**(1-2):99-104

[127] Yamamoto T, Saatcioglu F, Matsuda T. Cross-talk between bone morphogenic proteins and estrogen receptor signaling. Endocrinology. 2002;**143**(7):2635-2642

[128] Wang D, Huang P, Zhu B, Sun L, Huang Q, Wang J. Induction of estrogen receptor alpha-36 expression by bone morphogenetic protein 2 in breast cancer cell lines. Molecular Medicine Reports. 2012;**6**(3):591-596

[129] Matsumoto Y, Otsuka F, Takano M, Mukai T, Yamanaka R, Takeda M, et al. Estrogen and glucocorticoid regulate osteoblast differentiation through the interaction of bone morphogenetic protein-2 and tumor necrosis factor-alpha in C2C12 cells. Molecular and Cellular Endocrinology. 2010;**325**(1-2):118-127

[130] Qian SW, Liu Y, Wang J, Nie JC, Wu MY, Tang Y, et al. BMP4 cross-talks with estrogen/ERalpha signaling to regulate adiposity and glucose metabolism in females. eBioMedicine. 2016;**11**:91-100

[131] Wang YC, Xiao XL, Li N, Yang D, Xing Y, Huo R, et al. Oestrogen inhibits BMP4-induced BMP4 expression in cardiomyocytes: A potential mechanism of oestrogen-mediated protection against cardiac hypertrophy. British Journal of Pharmacology. 2015;**172**(23):5586-5595

[132] Liu Y, Du SY, Ding M, Dou X, Zhang FF, Wu ZY, et al. The

BMP4-Smad signaling pathway regulates hyperandrogenism development in a female mouse model. The Journal of Biological Chemistry. 2017;**292**(28):11740-11750

[133] Giacomini D, Paez-Pereda M, Stalla J, Stalla GK, Arzt E. Molecular interaction of BMP-4, TGF-beta, and estrogens in lactotrophs: Impact on the PRL promoter. Molecular Endocrinology. 2009;**23**(7):1102-1114

[134] Serra M, Alysandratos KD, Hawkins F, McCauley KB, Jacob A, Choi J, et al. Pluripotent stem cell differentiation reveals distinct developmental pathways regulating lung- versus thyroid-lineage specification. Development. 2017;**144**(21):3879-3893

[135] Villacorte M, Delmarcelle AS, Lernoux M, Bouquet M, Lemoine P, Bolsee J, et al. Thyroid follicle development requires Smad1/5- and endothelial cell-dependent basement membrane assembly. Development. 2016;**143**(11):1958-1970

[136] Meng X, Zhu P, Li N, Hu J, Wang S, Pang S, et al. Expression of BMP-4 in papillary thyroid carcinoma and its correlation with tumor invasion and progression. Pathology, Research and Practice. 2017;**213**(4):359-363

[137] Conde SJ, Luvizotto Rde A, de Sibio MT, Nogueira CR. Thyroid hormone status interferes with estrogen target gene expression in breast cancer samples in menopausal women. ISRN Endocrinology. 2014;**2014**:317398

[138] Wang ZY, Yin L. Estrogen receptor alpha-36 (ER-alpha36): A new player in human breast cancer. Molecular and Cellular Endocrinology. 2015;**418**(Pt 3):193-206

[139] Deng H, Zhang XT, Wang ML, Zheng HY, Liu LJ, Wang ZY. ER-alpha36-mediated rapid estrogen signaling positively regulates ER-positive breast cancer stem/progenitor cells. PLoS One. 2014;**9**(2):e88034

[140] Wang Q, Jiang J, Ying G, Xie XQ, Zhang X, Xu W, et al. Tamoxifen enhances stemness and promotes metastasis of ERalpha36(+) breast cancer by upregulating ALDH1A1 in cancer cells. Cell Research. 2018;**28**(3):336-358

[141] Wang Z, Zhang X, Shen P, Loggie BW, Chang Y, Deuel TF. Identification, cloning, and expression of human estrogen receptor-alpha36, a novel variant of human estrogen receptor-alpha66. Biochemical and Biophysical Research Communications. 2005;**336**(4):1023-1027

[142] Lee LM, Cao J, Deng H, Chen P, Gatalica Z, Wang ZY. ER-alpha36, a novel variant of ER-alpha, is expressed in ER-positive and -negative human breast carcinomas. Anticancer Research. 2008;**28**(1B):479-483

[143] Omarjee S, Jacquemetton J, Poulard C, Rochel N, Dejaegere A, Chebaro Y, et al. The molecular mechanisms underlying the ERalpha-36-mediated signaling in breast cancer. Oncogene. 2017;**36**(18):2503-2514

[144] Lin SL, Yan LY, Zhang XT, Yuan J, Li M, Qiao J, et al. ER-alpha36, a variant of ER-alpha, promotes tamoxifen agonist action in endometrial cancer cells via the MAPK/ERK and PI3K/Akt pathways. PLoS One. 2010;**5**(2):e9013

[145] Wang X, Jiang SW, Wang L, Sun Y, Xu F, He H, et al. Interfering effects of bisphenol A on in vitro growth of preantral follicles and maturation of oocyes. Clinica Chimica Acta. 2018;**485**:119-125

[146] Watson CS, Bulayeva NN, Wozniak AL, Finnerty CC. Signaling from the membrane via membrane estrogen receptor-alpha: Estrogens,

xenoestrogens, and phytoestrogens. Steroids. 2005;**70**(5-7):364-371

[147] Thent ZC, Froemming GRA, Muid S. Bisphenol A exposure disturbs the bone metabolism: An evolving interest towards an old culprit. Life Sciences. 2018;**198**:1-7

[148] Mei J, Hu H, McEntee M, Plummer H 3rd, Song P, Wang HC. Transformation of non-cancerous human breast epithelial cell line MCF10A by the tobacco-specific carcinogen NNK. Breast Cancer Research and Treatment. 2003;**79**(1):95-105

[149] Dreier DA, Connors KA, Brooks BW. Comparative endpoint sensitivity of in vitro estrogen agonist assays. Regulatory Toxicology and Pharmacology. 2015;**72**(2):185-193

[150] Huang R, Sakamuru S, Martin MT, Reif DM, Judson RS, Houck KA, et al. Profiling of the Tox21 10K compound library for agonists and antagonists of the estrogen receptor alpha signaling pathway. Scientific Reports. 2014;**4**:5664

[151] Peyre L, Rouimi P, de Sousa G, Helies-Toussaint C, Carre B, Barcellini S, et al. Comparative study of bisphenol A and its analogue bisphenol S on human hepatic cells: A focus on their potential involvement in nonalcoholic fatty liver disease. Food and Chemical Toxicology: An International Journal Published for the British Industrial Biological Research Association. 2014;**70**:9-18

[152] Eladak S, Grisin T, Moison D, Guerquin MJ, N'Tumba-Byn T, Pozzi-Gaudin S, et al. A new chapter in the bisphenol A story: Bisphenol S and bisphenol F are not safe alternatives to this compound. Fertility and Sterility. 2015;**103**(1):11-21

[153] Rochester JR, Bolden AL. Bisphenol S and F: A systematic review and comparison of the hormonal activity of Bisphenol A substitutes. Environmental Health Perspectives. 2015;**123**(7):643-650

[154] Williams GP, Darbre PD. Low-dose environmental endocrine disruptors, increase aromatase activity, estradiol biosynthesis and cell proliferation in human breast cells. Molecular and Cellular Endocrinology. 2019;**486**:55-64

[155] Katagiri T, Watabe T. Bone morphogenetic proteins. Cold Spring Harbor Perspectives in Biology. 2016;**8**(6)

[156] Pupo M, Pisano A, Lappano R, Santolla MF, De Francesco EM, Abonante S, et al. Bisphenol A induces gene expression changes and proliferative effects through GPER in breast cancer cells and cancer-associated fibroblasts. Environmental Health Perspectives. 2012;**120**(8):1177-1182

[157] Song H, Zhang T, Yang P, Li M, Yang Y, Wang Y, et al. Low doses of bisphenol A stimulate the proliferation of breast cancer cells via ERK1/2/ERRgamma signals. Toxicology in Vitro. 2015;**30**(1 Pt B):521-528

[158] Kuukasjarvi T, Kononen J, Helin H, Holli K, Isola J. Loss of estrogen receptor in recurrent breast cancer is associated with poor response to endocrine therapy. Journal of Clinical Oncology. 1996;**14**(9):2584-2589

[159] Le Romancer M, Poulard C, Cohen P, Sentis S, Renoir JM, Corbo L. Cracking the estrogen receptor's posttranslational code in breast tumors. Endocrine Reviews. 2011;**32**(5):597-622

[160] Lapensee EW, Tuttle TR, Fox SR, Ben-Jonathan N. Bisphenol A at low nanomolar doses confers chemoresistance in estrogen receptor-alpha-positive and -negative breast

cancer cells. Environmental Health Perspectives. 2009;**117**(2):175-180

[161] Huang B, Luo N, Wu X, Xu Z, Wang X, Pan X. The modulatory role of low concentrations of bisphenol A on tamoxifen-induced proliferation and apoptosis in breast cancer cells. Environmental Science and Pollution Research International. 2019;**26**(3):2353-2362

[162] Riggins RB, Lan JP, Zhu Y, Klimach U, Zwart A, Cavalli LR, et al. ERRgamma mediates tamoxifen resistance in novel models of invasive lobular breast cancer. Cancer Research. 2008;**68**(21):8908-8917

[163] Gu W, Dong N, Wang P, Shi C, Yang J, Wang J. Tamoxifen resistance and metastasis of human breast cancer cells were mediated by the membrane-associated estrogen receptor ER-alpha36 signaling in vitro. Cell Biology and Toxicology. 2017;**33**(2):183-195

[164] Shee K, Jiang A, Varn FS, Liu S, Traphagen NA, Owens P, et al. Cytokine sensitivity screening highlights BMP4 pathway signaling as a therapeutic opportunity in ER(+) breast cancer. The FASEB Journal. 2019;**33**(2):1644-1657

[165] Welte T, Zhang XH, Rosen JM. Repurposing antiestrogens for tumor immunotherapy. Cancer Discovery. 2017;**7**(1):17-19

[166] Lin Z, Zhang X, Zhao F, Ru S. Bisphenol S promotes the cell cycle progression and cell proliferation through ERalpha-cyclin D-CDK4/6-pRb pathway in MCF-7 breast cancer cells. Toxicology and Applied Pharmacology. 2019;**366**:75-82

[167] Huang W, Zhao C, Zhong H, Zhang S, Xia Y, Cai Z. Bisphenol S induced epigenetic and transcriptional changes in human breast cancer cell line MCF-7. Environmental Pollution. 2019;**246**:697-703

[168] Gayrard V, Lacroix MZ, Grandin FC, Collet SH, Mila H, Viguie C, et al. Oral systemic bioavailability of Bisphenol A and Bisphenol S in pigs. Environmental Health Perspectives. 2019;**127**(7):77005

Chapter 3

A Novel SASH1-IQGAP1-E-Cadherin Signal Cascade Mediates Breast Cancer Metastasis

Ding'an Zhou, Xing Zeng, Yadong Li, Zhixiong Wu and Xin Wan

Abstract

SAM and SH3 domain-containing protein 1 (SASH1) was previously described as a candidate tumor suppressor gene in breast cancer and colon cancer to mediate tumor metastasis and tumor growth. However, the underlying mechanism that SASH1 implements breast cancer metastasis in most solid cancers remains unexplored. In this study, SASH1 was identified to bind to IQ motif-containing GTPase activating protein 1 (IQGAP1). In breast cancer tissues, there was a correlation between the expressions of SASH1 and IQGAP1 ($P < 0.05$), and the expressions of SASH1 and IQGAP1 proteins were, respectively, correlated with the expression of E-cadherin ($P < 0.001$). In addition, the expressions of SASH1 and IQGAP1 proteins were correlated with tumor diameter and tumor grade (all $P < 0.05$) but without lymph node metastasis ($P > 0.05$). Therefore, it is suggested that SASH1 may form a new signaling cascade with IQGAP1 and E-cadherin to regulate breast cancer metastasis.

Keywords: breast neoplasms, gene expression regulation, cadherins, SAM and SH3 domain-containing protein 1 (SASH1), IQ motif-containing GTPase activating protein 1 (IQGAP1)

1. Introduction

Breast neoplasm is the most common cancer in women, which is originated from mammary epithelial tissue. The age of breast cancer is about 40–60 years old or before and after menopause. The morbidity of breast cancer is showed to be an upward trend year by year [1]. There are many factors that trigger breast cancer; however, the genetic factors only account for 10 and 90% of inducing factors of breast cancer remain to be investigated. SASH1 is a novel tumor suppressor gene, which is located in chromosome 6q24.3 [2] and is expressed in most of human tissues and cells except for lymphocytes and dendritic cells [3]. SASH1 was originally identified as a candidate tumor suppressor gene in breast cancer and colon cancer, regulating tumorigenesis of breast and other solid cancers and the adhesive and migratory behavior of cancer cells in tumor formation [4, 5]. Compared with that in normal breast epithelial tissues, SASH1 is downregulated in 74% of epithelial tissues of breast cancer-affected individuals [4, 6]. Some studies indicate that SASH1 downregulation is associated with tumor metastasis [3, 5]. Other studies indicate downregulated SASH1 promotes metastasis of hepatoma carcinoma cells through Shh signal pathway [7].

IQGAP1 is a scaffolding protein with 189 kDa of molecule weight, which contains multiple protein-interacting domains, such as a calponin homology domain, a polyproline-binding domain, four calmodulin-binding motifs, and a Ras GAP-related domain [8, 9]. The binding players of IQGAP1 proteins are involved in actin, calmodulin, members of the Rho GTPase family (i.e., Rac1 and Cdc42), Rap1, E-cadherin, β-catenin, members of the mitogen-activated protein kinase (MAPK) pathway, and adenomatous polyposis coli [8, 10]. Various basic cellular activities such as cytoskeletal organization, cell-cell adhesion, cell migration, transcription, and signal transduction are mediated by the bindings of IQGAP1 to these proteins [11]. Cell-cell adhesion of epithelial cells is predominantly mediated by E-cadherin and the associated catenin complex [12], which includes α-catenin (102 kDa), β-catenin (92 kDa), and γ-catenin/plakoglobin (83 kDa). β-Catenin combines with E-cadherin, and α-catenin links this E-cadherin/β-catenin complex to the actin cytoskeleton, which is essential for E-cadherin to express its full adhesive function. Remodeling of this adhesive sequence leads to cell detachment or loosening of cell-cell contact, which promotes epithelial cells to move as clusters, and IQGAP1 is involved in the remodeling of the adhesive complexes of epithelial cells [11, 13–15]. Our previous studies suggest that SASH1 is associated with MAP2K2 to cross talk with ERK1/2-CREB cascade to trigger melanin synthesis in the formation of hyperpigmentation plaques of a kind of dyschromatosis [16]. Importantly, our previous studies also indicate that SASH1 not only bind to G alpha S protein (Gαs) but IQGAP1 to form a novel Gαs-SASH1-IQGAP1-E-cadherin cascade and mutated SASH1(s) which mediate E-cadherin expression through the Gαs-SASH1-IQGAP1-E-cadherin cascade to promote directional migration of melanocytes or melanoma cells [17]. So, it is speculated that this mechanism may also exist in breast cancer cells. Taken above, the associations between SASH1 and IQGAP1 in breast cancer cells and the expression of SASH1, IQGAP1, and E-cadherin were analyzed by immunohistochemistry analyses in 80 cases of the affected individuals of breast cancer. Furthermore, the expression relationship among SASH1, IQGAP1, and E-cadherin and the associations between clinical index of breast cancer patients and the expression of SASH1 and IQGAP1, respectively, were assessed to find out novel interference targets for early prevention of breast cancer metastasis.

2. Material and methods

2.1 Plasmid construction of HA-IQGAP1-pcDNA3.0 and pEGFP-C3-SASH1

The construction of pEGFP-C3-SASH1 recombined vectors was mainly referred to our previous description [17]. IQGAP1 cDNA was obtained from Han Jiahuai Lab, Xiamen University (Xiamen, Fujian, China), and cloned into pcDNA3.0-HA vector. PCR was performed with IQGAP1 cDNA as template using TransTaq® DNA Polymerase High Fidelity (TransGen Biotech, Ltd., Beijing, China) using the following cloning primers of IQGAP1: sense primer, 5'-TAGTCTAGAAT GTCCG CCGCAACGAG-3'(Xba I inserted) and antisense primer, 5′-CCGCTCGAGTTACTTCCCGTAGAACTTTTTG-3′ (Xho I inserted). The amplification conditions were as follows: 95°C 2 min, 95°C 30 s, 58°C 30 s, and 72°C 1 min for 30 cycles and 72°C 5 min and 4°C forever. The recombined vectors were identified by enzyme digestion of endonuclease and CDS of SASH1 and IQGAP1 genes.

2.2 Cell culture and transfection

Human breast cancer cell lines including SK-BR-3 cells were obtained from the Cell Bank of Chinese Academy of Sciences (Shanghai, China). After several times of passage, cells were used and cultured in Dulbecco's Modified Eagle's medium (DMEM) (Gibco, Logan, UT), containing 10% BI fetal bovine serum (Bioind, Israel) and 1% penicillin-streptomycin solution at 37°C with 5% CO_2. SK-BR-3 cells were subcultured for three times and cultured to logarithmic growth phase for plasmid transfection. The HA-IQGAP1-pcDNA3.0 and pEGFP-C3-SASH1 were transfected into SK-BR-3 cells according to different combinations using PEI prepared by us. The transfected SK-BR-3 cells were divided into three groups, that is, two single-vector transfection groups and one double-vector transfection group. At 48 h after transfection, the transfected SK-BR-3 cells were lysed and collected for immunoprecipitation assays.

2.3 Immunoprecipitation and immunoblotting

Transfected SK-BR-3 cells were gently washed in PBS three times and then lysed for 25 min using IP-WB lysis buffer (Beyondtime Inc. Ltd., Jiangsu, China) with complete protease inhibitor cocktail per 10-cm dish for 20 min on ice. The cell lysates were transferred to 1.5 ml microcentrifuge tubes. The extracts were centrifuged for 15 min at 12,000 rpm at 4°C. The supernatants were immunoprecipitated using GFP mouse monoclonal antibody (T0005, Affinity Biosciences, Cincinnati, OH, USA) or HA mouse monoclonal antibody (mAb) (Abmart, Shanghai, China) as performed in our previous descriptions [17]. The immunoprecipitates were washed with PBS for three times and subjected to western blotting as previously described [16, 17]. Most of the western blots were mainly performed in our previous reports [17]. The associated HA-IQGAP1 or GFP-SASH1 was detected by western blot along with β-tubulin as loading control. The primary antibodies used in western blot were as follows: anti-GFP, anti-HA, and anti-β-tubulin (10B1) mouse mAb (EarthOx Life Science, Millbrae, CA, USA or Shanghai Genomics, Shanghai, China).

2.4 Clinical cases

All breast cancer patients who underwent surgery were followed by treatment in accordance with the National Comprehensive Cancer Network clinical practice guidelines. Fresh primary breast cancer tissues and some of the corresponding adjacent tissues were collected from 80 breast ductal carcinoma patients undergoing resection from May 2015 to June 2016 at the Chongqing Cancer Hospital. Histological diagnosis and tumor-node-metastasis staging of cancer were determined in accordance with the American Joint Committee on Cancer manual criteria for breast cancer. Written informed consent regarding tissue and data used for scientific purposes was obtained from all participating patients. The study was approved by the Research Ethics Committees of the affiliated Hospitals of Guizhou Medical University and Chongqing Cancer Hospital. All of the breast cancer cases were diagnosed by pathological examinations (HE staining and immunohistochemistry analyses). In the clinical cases of breast cancer, 26 cases are with lymph node metastasis, 51 cases are without lymph node metastasis, and 3 cases could not acquire the information of lymph node metastasis. Breast tumor diameters of 16 cases were <1 cm, those of 41 cases were 1.1–2 cm, those of 18 cases were 2.1–3 cm, and those of 5 cases were >3 cm. According to WHO histological classification of breast tumors (2003), 80 cases of breast invasive ductal carcinoma were graded histologically in terms of duct formation, nuclear pleomorphism, and mitosis. Among the 80 cases of breast invasive ductal carcinoma, 65 cases were graded into 3 grades: 8 cases belonged to grade I, 47 cases to grade II, and 10 cases to grade III.

2.5 Immunohistochemical analyses of SASH1, IQGAP1, and E-cadherin

The breast cancer tissues obtained from surgical operation were fixed at 4°C in 10% formaldehyde solution for 24 h. The excess fat and other tissues of breast cancer tissues were removed and embedded with paraffin and made into 5 millimeter (mm) tissue sections. The tissue sections (5 mm) were baked at 56°C and dehydrated and subjected to peroxidase blocking. Tissues of human breast cancer and corresponding adjacent tissues were immunohistochemically stained with SASH1 rabbit polyclonal antibody (pAb) (A302-265A-1, Bethyl Laboratories, Inc., Texas, USA, or Novus Biologicals, USA), IQGAP1 rabbit polyclonal antibody (Bethyl Laboratories, Inc., Texas, USA), and E-Cadherin (24E10) Rabbit mAb (#3195, Cell Signaling Technology). Primary antibodies were added and incubated at 37°C and then for overnight at 4°C. After washing three times for 10 min each with TBS, the sections were incubated with horseradish peroxidase-conjugated anti-rabbit and anti-mouse universal secondary antibodies for 30 min at 37°C. Subsequently, the sections were counterstained with hematoxylin mounted, observed, and photographed under the positive position microscope BX51 at a 100× magnification or a 400× magnification. Finally, the stained slides were observed under a microscope, and images were acquired [17]. The experimental protocols were mainly referred to our previous description [17].

According to the staining intensity of tumor cells, the three proteins, SASH1, IQGAP1, and E-cadherin, were scored and divided into four grades: 0 score (−), 1 score (+), 2 score (++), and 3 score (+++). The three proteins were also scored according to positive cells' percentage of the three proteins and divided into six grades: 0 score (<1%), 1 score (1–20%), 2 score (21–40%), 3 score (41–60%), 4 score (61–80%), 5 score (81–100%). Based on the staining intensity of SASH1, IQGAP1, and E-cadherin, the staining intensity and positive cells' percentage of three proteins were calculated as in our previous description [16]. Total scores of each visual field were determined by the formula: staining intensity scores of positive cells × scores of positive cells' percentage = total scores of each view fields.

2.6 Statistical analyses

All of experimental results were repeated for three times and statistically analyzed using SPSS 16.0 statistical software. Chi square test was performed to analyze the IHC results of breast cancer tissues and the relationship between expression of SASH1 and IQGAP1 and clinical indicators. Rank-sum test was used to assess the grading relationship between the SASH1 and E-cadherin and IQGAP1 and E-cadherin, respectively. Spearman correlation coefficient method was used to assess the correlation between expressed scores of SASH1 and E-cadherin and IQGAP1 and E-cadherin, respectively. The data are indicated as mean ± standard error of the mean (SEM), and the difference was statistically significant with $P < 0.05$. Cartograms were plotted with GraphPad Prism 5.

3. Results

3.1 SASH1 is associated with IQGAP1

To identify the associations between SASH1 and IQGAP1, HA-IQGAP1-pcDNA3.0 and pEGFP-C3-SASH1 were constructed and were singly or combinedly transfected into SK-BR-3 cells and immunoprecipitation; western blot (IP-WB) was performed to identify the associations between exogenous SASH1 and exogenous IQGAP1. HA-IQGAP1 and GFP-SASH1 were singly or in pair transfected into SK-BR-3 cells at 48 h posttransfection, the transfected cells were lysed, and HA-IQGAP1 was immunoprecipitated, and the associated GFP-SASH1 was detected by GFP antibody. The associated HA-IQGAP1 and GFP-SASH1 in the immunoprecipitates and cell lysates (input) were confirmed by western blot. Meanwhile, GFP-SASH1 and HA-IQGAP1 were also either single or in pair transfected into SK-BR-3 cells and after 48 h of transfection, the transfected cells were lysed and were GFP-SASH1 was immunoprecipitated and the associated HA-IQGAP1 was detected by HA antibody. The associated GFP-SASH1 and HA-IQGAP1 in the immunoprecipitates and cell lysates (input) were identified by western blot. Finally, our IP-WB analyses confirmed that exogenous SASH1 was associated with exogenous IQGAP1 (**Figure 1**).

3.2 There was a positive correlation between SASH1 and IQGAP1 expression in breast cancer tissues

IHC analyses confirmed that the positive staining of SASH1 and IQGAP1 protein was light brown in breast cancer tissues, the cell nucleus was purple, and the distribution of SASH1 and IQGAP1 was located in the same sites of breast cancer tissues. SASH1 and IQGAP1 show the same or similar expression tendency in breast cancer tissues, i.e., low level of SASH1 expression is followed by low level of IQGAP1 expression and high expression of SASH1 is accompanied by high expression of IQGAP1 (**Figure 2A**). A total of 80 breast cancer tissues were divided into four groups according to the median value of SASH1 and IQGAP1 protein expression scores: SASH1 scores <1.23 were considered as low expression, SASH1 scores ≥1.23 were considered as high expression, IQGAP1 scores <0.78 were maintained as low expression, and SASH1 scores ≥0.78 were maintained as high expression. Statistical analyses indicated that in the 80 cases of breast cancer tissues, cases with low SASH1 expression accounted for 56.3% (45/80) and the cases with low IQGAP1 expression were more than those of high IQGAP1

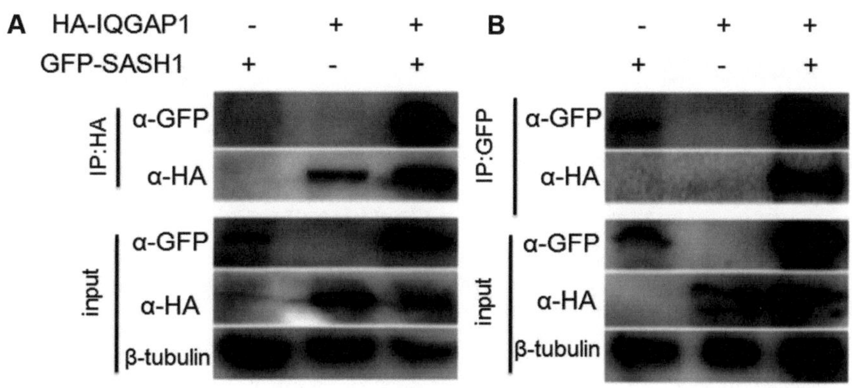

Figure 1.
SASH1 is associated with IQGAP1. (A) GFP-SASH1 and HA-IQGAP1 were singly or in pair transfected into SK-BR-3 cells, and at 36 h after transfection, the transfected cells were lysed and collected for IP-WB analyses. HA-IQGAP1 was immunoprecipitated, and the associated GFP-SASH1 was detected by western blot using GFP antibody. GFP-SASH1 and HA-IQGAP1 in the cell lysates (input) were detected by western blot along with β-tubulin with loading control. (B) HA-IQGAP1 and GFP-SASH1 were singly or in pair transfected into SK-BR-3 cells, and at 36 h after transfection, the transfected cells were lysed and collected for IP-WB analyses. GFP-SASH1 was immunoprecipitated, and the associated GFP-SASH1 was detected by western blot using GFP antibody. HA-IQGAP1 and GFP-SASH1 in the cell lysates (input) were analyzed by western blot along with β-tubulin with loading control.

expression (>65%, P = 0.015) (**Figure 2B**). And statistical analyses also suggested that in the 80 cases of breast cancer tissues, cases with low IQGAP1 expression accounted for 58.8% (47/80) and the cases with low IQGAP1 expression were more than those of high IQGAP1 expression (>60%, P = 0.011) (**Figure 2B**). Meanwhile, the IHC detection results of SASH1 and IQGAP1 were scored and analyzed by Spearman correlation analyses, and the scores of SASH1 and IQGAP1 were plotted by GraphPad Prism 5 software. In 80 cases of breast cancer tissues, except for 5 cases, SASH1 scores and IQGAP1 scores in most of cases closely

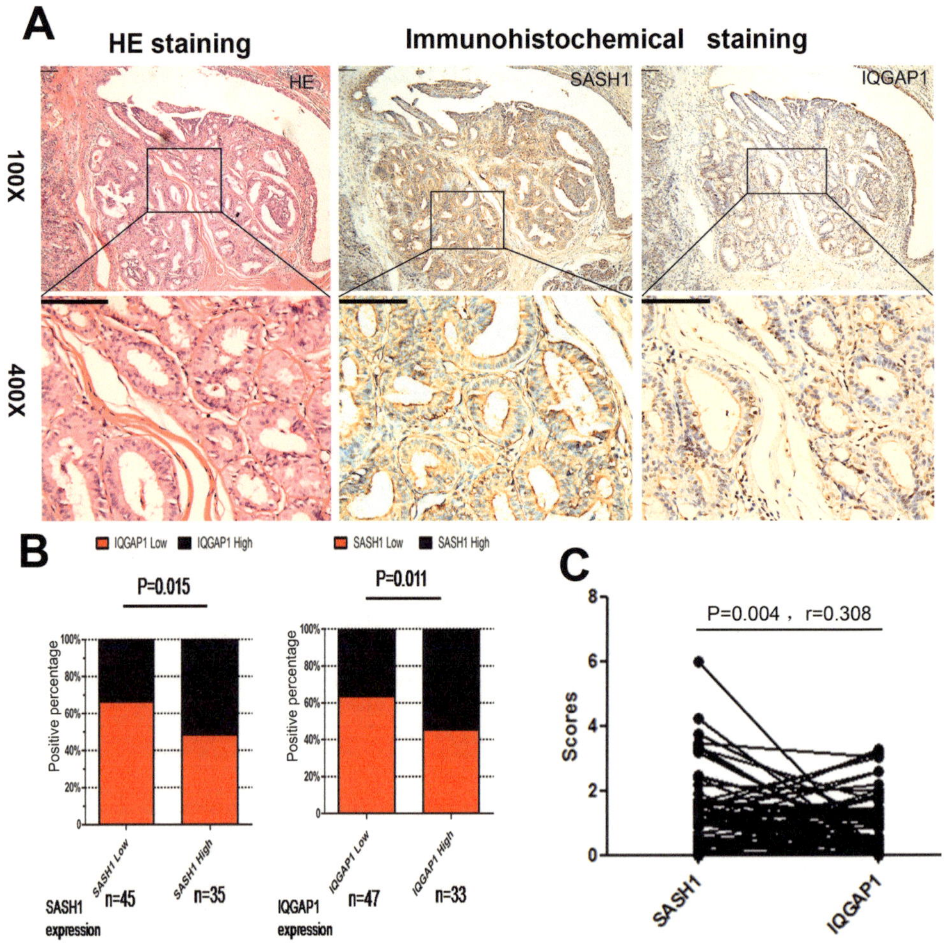

Figure 2.
SASH1 expression in 80 cases of breast cancer tissues which is positively correlated with IQGAP1. (A) The expressions of SASH1 and IQGAP1 in 80 cases of breast cancer tissues were detected by immunohistochemical staining method. The cell nucleus was dyed purple and SASH1 and IQGAP1 were dyed pale brown. The left panels were HE staining, and the middle panels and the right panels were IHC staining of SASH1 and IQGAP1. The figures in upper panels were 100× magnification, and one region in the 100× magnification figures was amplified for 400× and framed in black and showed in the bottom panels. (B) The expressions of SASH1 and IQGAP1 were scored, and the score results of SASH1 and IQGAP1 were plotted with GraphPad Prism 5 and analyzed by χ^2 test. The analysis results of SASH1 and IQGAP1 expressions in the left panel indicated that when SASH1 expression was low, the positive percentage of low expressed IQGAP1 was much more than that of high expressed IQGAP1. The expression of SASH1 showed significantly positive correlation with that of IQGAP1 (P = 0.015). And the statistical analyses also suggested that when IQGAP1 expression was low, the positive percentage of low expressed SASH1 was much more than that of high expressed SASH1. The expression of IQGAP1 demonstrated significantly positive correlation with that of SASH1 (P = 0.011). (C) The expressions of SASH1 and IQGAP1 were scored, and the score results of SASH1 and IQGAP1 were plotted with GraphPad Prism 5 and analyzed by Spearman correlation coefficient analyses. Spearman correlation coefficient analyses indicated that except for two score values of SASH1, expression of SASH1 and IQGAP1 showed good similar or same tendency of changes (P = 0.004).

intersected, which indicated that the SASH1 expression and IQGAP1 expression showed significantly positive correlation (r = 0.308, P = 0.004) (**Figure 2C**).

3.3 The expression of SASH1 and IQGAP1 protein in breast cancer was significantly correlated with tumor size and tumor grade

It has been known that the expression of SASH1 and IQGAP1 is associated with tumor metastasis. So, in this study, we further identify the relationship of expression of SASH1 and IQGAP1 with clinical data of breast cancer-affected individuals. Our analyses (**Table 1**) indicated that in 77 cases of breast cancer with lymph node dissection, the low expression rate of SASH1 protein in lymph node metastasis positive group was slightly higher than that in lymph node metastasis negative group. The low

Clinical parameters	Total	SASH1		IQGAP1		P
		Low	High	Low	High	
Lymph node metastasis[a]						>0.05
Positive	26	17	9	15	11	
Negative	51	28	23	30	21	
Tumor diameter/cm[b]						<0.05
≤1	16	8	8	10	6	
1.1–2	41	24	17	23	18	
2.1–3	18	9	9	10	8	
>3	5	4	1	4	1	
Histological grade[c]						<0.01
I	8	4	4	6	2	
II	47	26	21	24	23	
III	10	7	3	7	3	

[a]*N = 77.*
[b]*N = 80.*
[c]*N = 65.*

Table 1.
Association of SASH1 and IQGAP1 expressions with the clinical parameters of breast cancer patients (n).

E-cadherin	SASH1					IQGAP1				
	–	+	++	++	Total[a]	–	+	++	+++	Total[b]
–	4	6	6	1	17	8	8	1	0	17
+	6	20	2	0	28	12	12	4	0	28
++	5	25	3	0	33	12	19	2	0	33
+++	1	0	1	0	2	1	1	0	0	2
Total	16	51	12	1	80	33	40	7	0	80

[a]*r = 0.461, P < 0.001.*
[b]*r = 0.454, P < 0.001; by rank-sum test.*

Table 2.
Correlation of SASH1 and IQGAP1 expressions with E-cadherin expression rankin breast cancer tissues (n, N = 80).

expression rate of IQGAP1 protein was slightly lower than that of the negative lymph node metastasis group, but the difference was not statistically significant (65.4% vs. 54.9%, 57.7% vs. 58.8%, all P value > 0.05). In 80 cases of breast cancer, the low expression rate of SASH1 protein was 50.0, 58.5, 50.0, and 80.0%, respectively, in patients with tumor diameter <1.0 cm, 1.1–2.0 cm, 2.1–3.0 cm, and >3.0 cm. The low expression rates of IQGAP1 protein were 62.5, 56.1, 55.6, and 80.0%, respectively. There were significant differences between the two groups (P < 0.05). In 65 cases of breast cancer with histological grading data, the low expression rates of SASH1 protein in histological grading I, II, and III were 50.0, 55.3, and 70.0%, respectively. The low expression rates of IQGAP1 protein were 75.0, 51.1, and 70.0%, respectively. There were significant differences between groups (P < 0.01).

3.4 The expression of SASH1 and IQGAP1 is positively related with E-cadherin, respectively, in breast cancer tissues

SASH1 and IQGAP1 have been identified to be involved in tumor metastasis. And immunohistochemistry (IHC) analyses were performed to detect the expression of E-cadherin in breast cancer tissues and the relevance of E-cadherin with SASH1 and IQGAP1, respectively. IHC analyses indicated that E-cadherin was mainly located in the cytoplasma membrane of breast cancer tissues. According to the positive intensity of E-cadherin staining, E-cadherin protein expression in breast cancer tissues was graded to four grades, and meanwhile the positive intensity of SASH1 protein staining was also graded to four grades. Statistical analyses suggested that expression of SASH1 protein was significantly positive related to that of E-cadherin (r = 0.461, P < 0.001 (**Table 2** and **Figure 3**)).

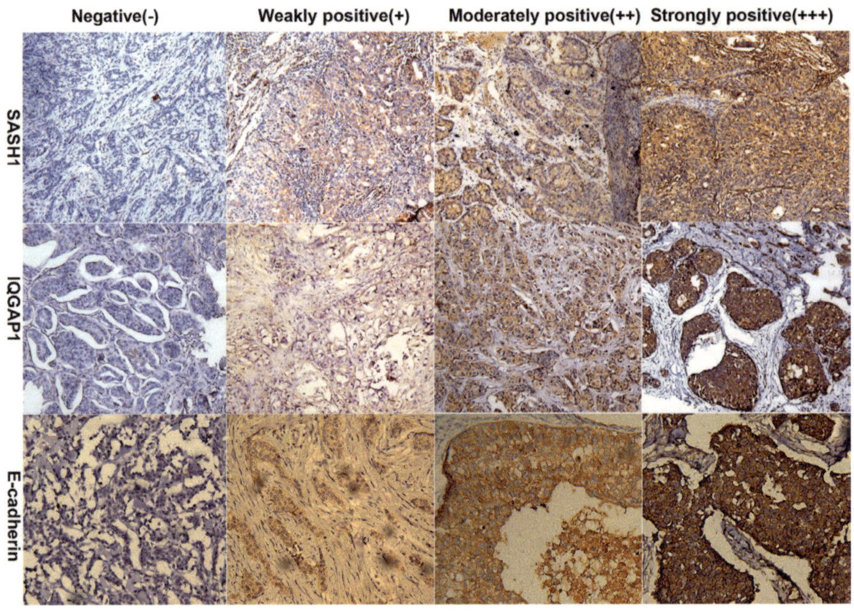

Figure 3.
SASH1, IQGAP1, and E-cadherin proteins showed consistent changes in the breast cancer tissues. The cell nucleus was dyed purple and SASH1, IQGAP1, and E-cadherin were dyed pale brown, and the magnification is 200×. According to staining intensity of tumor cells and the numbers of positive cells, the immunohistochemical results of SASH1, IQGAP1, and E-cadherin proteins were divided into four grades: negative (−), weakly positive (+), moderately positive (++), and strongly positive (+++). The expression of SASH1 was positively correlated with that of E-cadherin and the expression of IQGAP1 show positive correlation with that of E-cadherin. The cell nucleus was dyed purple, and SASH1, IQGAP1, and, E-cadherin were dyed pale brown, and the magnification is 200×.

SASH1 and E-cadherin staining intensity was moderately positive staining intensity, respectively, which was defined low expression. And further statistical analyses suggested SASH1 and E-cadherin were downregulated in 77 cases (77/80, 96.25%) of breast cancer tissues. All of these indicated that the low expression of SASH1 and the low expression of E-cadherin protein in breast cancer tissue are in good agreement.

According to the staining intensity of IQGAP1 protein and E-cadherin protein in 80 cases of breast cancer, the staining intensity of E-cadherin and IQGAP1 was divided into four grades. Statistical analyses demonstrated that expression of IQGAP1 protein was significantly positive related to that of E-cadherin ($r = 0.454$, $P < 0.001$ (**Table 2** and **Figure 3**)). Staining intensity of IQGAP1 and E-cadherin was moderately positive staining intensity, respectively, which was defined low expression. And further statistical analyses suggested IQGAP1 and E-cadherin were both downregulated in 78 cases (78/80, 97.5%) of breast cancer tissues. All of these indicated that the low expression of IQGAP1 and the low expression of E-cadherin showed better consistency in breast cancer tissue.

4. Conclusion

Clinical research indicates that occurrence of breast cancer is associated with many factors including genetic factors, environment, and lifestyle. SASH1, a tumor suppressor gene, is downregulated in most of neoplasms. Decrease or deletion of SASH1 expression is closely related to tumor metastasis [4, 5, 18]. It has been reported that the expression of SASH1 protein in osteosarcoma tissues with lung metastasis is significantly lower than that in osteosarcoma tissues without lung metastasis [19]. Upregulated SASH1 can significantly suppress the migration of cervical carcinoma Hela cells, and, in contrast, knockdown of SASH1 significantly results in reduced adhesion ability of human colon cancer SW480 cells and mouse rectal cancer CMT-93 cells and enhanced migration ability of these tumor cells [3]. Downregulation of SASH1 protein expression in thyroid tumor cells may play an important role in thyroid tumor metastasis [20]. SASH1 mRNA is downregulated in primary liver cancer and thyroid cancer [5]. Compared with corresponding normal tissues, SASH1 protein is downregulated in 37 cases among 50 cases of breast cancer tissues and SASH1 expression loss is associated with breast cancer metastasis [4]. All of these studies suggest that expression loss of SASH1 medicates tumor metastasis. In this study, our IHC analyses identified that in 80 cases of breast cancer tissues, low expression of SASH1 protein in 45 cases (45/80 56.3%) was found, which indicated that SASH1 was downregulated in breast cancer.

IQGAP1 proteins are members of the evolutionarily conserved scaffolding protein family and are more widely expressed than other members of the family [21, 22]. IQGAP1 interacts with specific proteins such as actin, calmodulin, Rho GTPase family members, E-cadherin, and β-catenin. The interactions of IQGAP1 with those specific proteins medicate multiple cell activities such as cell scaffold, intercellular adhesion, metastasis, invasion, transcription, and cell signal transduction. For example, the binding of IQGAP1 to β-catenin to form E-cadherin/β-catenin complex inhibits intercellular adhesion of epithelial cells and promotes β-catenin-mediated transcriptional activation [9]. IQGAP1 protein ,which mediates E-cadherin-mediated-intercellular adhesion, is the key molecule in cell polarization and directed migration [23]. IQGAP1 expression is showed to be of prognostic significance in advanced colorectal carcinoma, and a shorter overall survival of colorectal carcinoma patients can be predicted by diffuse expression pattern of IQGAP1 [11]. In this study, IHC analyses indicated, in 80 cases of breast cancer tissues, IQGAP1 protein level was significantly low in 47 cases accounting for 58.8%, which suggested that IQGAP1 was downregulated in breast cancer.

Multiple endocrine neoplasia type 1 (MEN1) is a dominantly inherited tumor syndrome that results from the mutation of the MEN1 gene that encodes protein menin. MEN1 is revealed to bind to IQGAP1 and increases E-cadherin/β-catenin interaction with IQGAP1 and a novel menin-IQGAP1 pathway that controls cell migration and cell-cell adhesion found in endocrine cells [24]. Activated Rac1 and Cdc42 can bind to IQGAP1, and the bindings of IQGAP1 and Rac1 as well as Cdc42 promote cell mobility and polarization [25, 26]. IQGAP1 is both a downstream effector and an upstream activator of Cdc42, where active Cdc42 antagonizes IQGAP1 dissociation of the cell-cell contacts [27, 28]. Cdc42 inhibits IQGAP1's role in polarized secretion in β-cells or perhaps migration [29]. In this study, IP-WB analyses indicated the protein-protein interactions between SASH1 and IQGAP1. It has been reported that SASH1 expression suppresses cell proliferation and interacts with cytoskeletal proteins, which promotes cell matrix adhesion [3, 4]. Meanwhile, other studies have identified that SASH1 is associated with scaffold proteins and foster tumor migration [3]. Hence, we speculate that the bindings of SASH1 and IQGAP1 co-mediate breast cancer metastasis.

Recurrence or metastasis of breast cancer is the leading cause of breast cancer-related death. It has been identified that epithelial-mesenchymal transition (EMT) plays a pivotal role in tumor metastasis through generation and survival of induced circulating tumor cells [30]. One of the EMT functions is to downregulate and relocate the epithelial cell adhesion protein including the leading actor, E-cadherin [31]. The decreased expression of E-cadherin in breast cancer was associated with high pathological grade, tumor volume enlargement, lymph node metastasis, and distant metastasis and with disease rehabilitation and overall survival time, which indicates that reduced expression or function loss of E-cadherin promotes breast cancer invasion and migration [32]. A dynamic equilibrium of E-cadherin between the E-cadherin-β-catenin-α-catenin complex and the E-cadherin-β-catenin-IQGAP1 complex at sites of cell-cell contact is proposed. The ratio between these two complexes could determine the strength of adhesion [33]. Our previous study found that SASH1 mutations enhanced mutated SASH1 expression, however induced downregulation of E-cadherin in epithelial cells of skin [17]. So it is speculated that there is a connection between SASH1 and E-cadherin. In this study, SASH1 protein level is positively correlated with E-cadherin, and IQGAP1 protein level is also positively correlated with E-cadherin, which also identifies the connection between SASH1 and E-cadherin.

Taken above, we speculate that SASH1 may mediate breast cancer metastasis through a novel SASH1-IQGAP1-E-cadherin signal cascade. When SASH1 and IQGAP1 protein levels in breast cancer tissues and breast cancer cells were low, the protein levels of E-cadherin are also reduced, which causes the reduced cell adhesion ability, the tumor cell ability which is easy to fall off, the enhanced invasion, and the tumor cell metastasis ability to distance. The novel findings about SASH1 will become a novel target to treat breast cancer, which will be conducive to the precision and diversification of breast cancer treatment, effectively improving the prognosis of patients. In this study, we find that low protein levels of SASH1 and IQGAP1 are related to tumor size, and the reduced protein levels of SASH1 and IQGAP1 are associated with tumor grading, which provides a new reference for the rapid diagnosis of tumor grading and tumor size. And our findings on SASH1 and IQGAP1 provide a new and more intuitive basis for determining the operation plan and resection range, judging the curative effect of operation and early detection of tumor metastasis and recurrence. However, in this study we find that low expression levels of SASH1 and IQGAP1 are significantly not related to lymph node metastasis, which presumably can be related to a small sample size of breast cancer tissues. The relationship between SASH1 and IQGAP1 with lymph node metastasis needs to be further investigated.

Acknowledgements

We thank Central Laboratory at Yongchuan Hospital, Chongqing Medical University and Clinical Research Center, and the Affiliated Hospital, Guizhou Medical University for housing experiments. We thank Zhou Xin and Jiang Xiaoli of the Breast Disease Diagnosis and Treatment Center of Chongqing Cancer Hospital for their active help and cooperation in sample collection. This work was supported partly by the High Level Talent Introduction Project of Affiliated Hospital of Guizhou Medical University (grant numbers: 2018I-1 and I-2017-19) and Guizhou Provincial Science and Technology Department Project (grant number: Qian Ke He LH [2017] 7193). This work was supported by the Yongchuan Hospital Project, Chongqing Medical University (YJYJ201347), Chongqing Education Commission Project (KJ1400201), and Guizhou's Introduction Project of Million Talents.

Conflict of interest

No conflict between the authors.

Notes/thanks/other declarations

Notes: The chapter text was mainly referred to our article entitled as "SASH1-IQGAP1-E-cadherin signal cascade may regulate breast cancer metastasis" (Tumor. 2017;37(6):633–641) which we published in the Chinese Journal Tumor in June 2017. In this chapter, we rewrite the chapter text according to the suggestions of reviewers.

The figures and tables of this chapter were taken or reedited from the figures and tables of our published article entitled "SASH1-IQGAP1-E-cadherin signal cascade may regulate breast cancer."

Declarations

We thanks the Chinese Journal Tumor allow us reuse the Figures and tables in our article entitled as"SASH1-IQGAP1-E-cadherin signal cascade may regulate breast cancer metastasis" (Tumor, 2017, 37(6): 633~641) which were published in the Chinese Journal Tumor. We are allowed to reuse the Figures, Tables and Text of our article entitled as "SASH1-IQGAP1-E-cadherin signal cascade may regulate breast cancer" under the terms of the Creative Commons Attribution License (CC BY) without having to obtain permission provided that the original source of publication.

Acronyms and abbreviations

DMEM	Dulbecco's Modified Eagle's medium
EMT	epithelial-mesenchymal transition
Gαs	guanine nucleotide-binding protein subunit-alpha isoforms short
HE staining	hematoxylin and eosin staining
IHC	immunohistochemical
IQGAP1	IQ motif-containing GTPase activating protein 1
IP-WB	immunoprecipitation-western blot
PEI	polyethylenimine
pAb	polyclonal antibody
SASH1	SAM and SH3 domain-containing 1
SEMs	standard error of the means

Author details

Ding'an Zhou*, Xing Zeng, Yadong Li, Zhixiong Wu and Xin Wan
Clinical Research Center, The Affiliated Hospital, Guizhou Medical University, Guiyang, Guizhou, The People's Republic of China

*Address all correspondence to: 460318918@qq.com

References

[1] Zhang Z et al. Expression of CXCR4 and breast cancer prognosis: A systematic review and meta-analysis. BMC Cancer. 2014;**14**(1):49

[2] Sheyu L, Hui L, Junyu Z, et al. Promoter methylation assay of SASH 1 gene in breast cancer. Journal of BUON. 2013;**18**(4):891-898

[3] Martini M, Gnann A, Scheikl D, Holzmann B, Janssen KP. The candidate tumor suppressor SASH1 interacts with the actin cytoskeleton and stimulates cell-matrix adhesion. The International Journal of Biochemistry & Cell Biology. 2011;**43**(11):1630-1640

[4] Zeller C, Hinzmann B, Seitz S, Prokoph H, Burkhard-Goettges E, Fischer J, et al. SASH1: A candidate tumor suppressor gene on chromosome 6q24.3 is downregulated in breast cancer. Oncogene. 2003;**22**(19):2972-2983

[5] Rimkus C, Martini M, Friederichs J, Rosenberg R, Doll D, Siewert JR, et al. Prognostic significance of downregulated expression of the candidate tumour suppressor gene SASH1 in colon cancer. British Journal of Cancer. 2006;**95**(10):1419-1423

[6] Lin S et al. Effects of SASH1 on melanoma cell proliferation and apoptosis in vitro. Molecular Medicine Reports. 2012;**6**(6):1243-1248

[7] He P et al. Overexpression of SASH1 inhibits the proliferation, invasion, and EMT in hepatocarcinoma cells. Oncology Research. 2016;**24**(1):25-32

[8] Brown MD, Sacks DB. IQGAP1 in cellular signaling: Bridging the GAP. Trends in Cell Biology. 2006;**16**(5):242-249

[9] Jadeski L et al. IQGAP1 stimulates proliferation and enhances tumorigenesis of human breast epithelial cells. The Journal of Biological Chemistry. 2008;**283**(2):1008-1017

[10] Owen D, Campbell L, Littlefield K, Evetts KA, Li Z, Sacks DB, et al. The IQGAP1-Rac1 and IQGAP1-Cdc42 interactions: Interfaces differ between the complexes. The Journal of Biological Chemistry. 2008;**283**:1692-1704

[11] Hiroyuki Hayashi KN, Aoki M, Hamasaki M, Enatsu S, Yamauchi Y, Yamashita Y, et al. Overexpression of IQGAP1 in advanced colorectal cancer correlates with poor prognosis—Critical role in tumor invasion. International Journal of Cancer. 2010;**126**:2563-2574

[12] Beavon IR. The E-cadherin-catenin complex in tumour metastasis: Structure, function and regulation. European Journal of Cancer. 2000;**36**:1607-1620

[13] Kuroda S et al. Role of IQGAP1, a target of the small GTPases Cdc42 and Rac1, in regulation of E-cadherin-mediated cell-cell adhesion. Science. 1998;**281**(5378):832-835

[14] Fukata M et al. Involvement of IQGAP1, an effector of Rac1 and Cdc42 GTPases, in cell-cell dissociation during cell scattering. Molecular and Cellular Biology. 2001;**21**(6):2165-2183

[15] Shimao Y, Nabeshima K, Inoue T, Koono M. Complex formation of IQGAP1 with ecadherin/catenin during cohort migration of carcinoma cells. Its possible association with localized release from cell-cell adhesion. Virchows Archiv. 2002;**441**:124-132

[16] Zhou D et al. p53 regulates ERK1/2/CREB cascade via a novel SASH1/MAP2K2 crosstalk to induce hyperpigmentation. Journal of Cellular and Molecular Medicine. 2017;**21**(10):2465-2480

[17] Zhou D et al. SASH1 regulates melanocyte transepithelial migration through a novel Galphas-SASH1-IQGAP1-E-Cadherin dependent pathway. Cellular Signalling. 2013;**25**(6):1526-1538

[18] Tsatmali M, Ancans J, Yukitake J, Thody AJ. Skin POMC peptides: Their actions at the human MC-1 receptor and roles in the tanning response. Pigment Cell Research, 2000;**13**(Suppl 8):125-129

[19] Meng Q et al. SASH1 regulates proliferation, apoptosis, and invasion of osteosarcoma cell. Molecular and Cellular Biochemistry. 2013;**373**(1-2):201-210

[20] Sun D, Zhou R, Liu H, et al. SASH1 inhibits proliferation and invasion of thyroid cancer cells through PI3K/Akt signaling pathway. International Journal of Clinical and Experimental Pathology. 2015;**8**(10):12276-12283

[21] Briggs MW, Sacks DB. IQGAP1 proteins are integral components of cytoskeletal regulation. EMBO Reports. 2003;**4**(6):571-574

[22] Sanchez-Laorden B, Viros A, Marais R. Mind the IQGAP. Cancer Cell. 2013;**23**(6):715-717

[23] Noritake J et al. IQGAP1: A key regulator of adhesion and migration. Journal of Cell Science. 2005;**118** (Pt 10):2085-2092

[24] Jizhou Yan YY, Zhang H, King C, Kan H-M, Cai Y, Yuan CX, et al. Menin interacts with IQGAP1 to enhance intercellular adhesion of β cells. Oncogene. 2009;**28**(7):973-982

[25] Mataraza JM et al. IQGAP1 promotes cell motility and invasion. The Journal of Biological Chemistry. 2003;**278**(42):41237-41245

[26] Watanabe T et al. Interaction with IQGAP1 links APC to Rac1, Cdc42, and actin filaments during cell polarization and migration. Developmental Cell. 2004;**7**(6):871-883

[27] Fukata M et al. Cdc42 and Rac1 regulate the interaction of IQGAP1 with beta-catenin. The Journal of Biological Chemistry. 1999;**274**(37):26044-26050

[28] Lambert M, Choquet D, Mege RM. Dynamics of ligand-induced, Rac1-dependent anchoring of cadherins to the actin cytoskeleton. The Journal of Cell Biology. 2002;**157**(3):469-479

[29] Rittmeyer EN et al. A dual role for IQGAP1 in regulating exocytosis. Journal of Cell Science. 2008;**121** (Pt 3):391-403

[30] Tsai JH, Yang J. Epithelial-mesenchymal plasticity in carcinoma metastasis. Genes & Development. 2013;**27**(20):2192-2206

[31] Thiery JP. Epithelial-mesenchymal transitions in tumour progression. Nature Reviews. Cancer. 2002;**2**(6):442-454

[32] Memni H et al. E-cadherin genetic variants predict survival outcome in breast cancer patients. Journal of Translational Medicine. 2016;**14**(1):320

[33] Takeuchi H et al. c-MET expression level in primary colon cancer: a predictor of tumor invasion and lymph node metastases. Clinical Cancer Research. 2003;**9**(4):1480-1488

Chapter 4

Evidence of BK_{Ca} Channelopathy-Driven Breast Cancer Metastasis to Brain

Divya Khaitan and Nagendra Ningaraj

Abstract

KCNMA1 encodes the a-subunit of the large conductance, voltage and Ca^{2+}-activated and Voltage-dependent potassium channel (BK_{Ca}) and was shown by others and us to be a potential drug target gene in several cancers, including breast cancer. In addition, we studied the role of alternative pre-mRNA splicing events of *KCNMA1* in migration, invasion, proliferation and dispersal of breast cancer cells. It is conceivable that by targeting gene variants we can attenuate processes such as distant metastasis and angiogenesis. Here we reviewed literature on the alternative splicing events specific to breast cancer metastasis to brain, its microenvironment, the biological activity of most alternatively spliced isoforms. We conclude that based on our and others' work *KCNMA1* and other such gene variants contribute to breast cancer dispersion, invasion, growth, and progression in the tumor micro-environment. Thus *KCNMA1*/BK_{Ca} channels and their variants are opportunistic diagnostic, prognostic and treatment targets in breast cancer.

Keywords: *KCNMA1* pre-mRNA splicing, BK_{Ca} channelopathy, breast cancer-dispersion, invasion, growth, angiogenesis, progression, treatment target

1. Introduction

1.1 Metastatic breast cancer etiology

Breast cancer is the most common type of cancer affecting women. Despite great advances in primary breast cancer treatment a significant number of women develop metastases in different organs of the body, especially brain [1], possibly as a result of the emergence of targeted and aggressive systemic cancer therapy. The actual incidence of brain metastases is not precisely known; however, studies suggest that 6–16% of patients with metastatic breast cancer develop brain metastases during their lifetime. Furthermore, autopsy studies have reported brain metastases in 18–30% of patients dying of breast cancer [2]. The majority of women who develop brain metastases have undergone aggressive treatment for stage IV disease [3–5]. Although brain metastasis is the leading cause of breast cancer death, its pathogenesis is poorly understood and the predictors of breast metastasis to brain are yet to be characterized. Albeit recent studies found genes that mediate breast cancer metastasis to brain [6, 7]. Targeting metastatic breast cancer cells in brain is extremely difficult as brain provides a "safe haven" for cancer cells. Gene expression profiling has been used to predict metastatic gene-expression signature that is present in a subset of primary breast tumors [8]. However, a reliable profile has not yet been identified that specifically predicts brain metastases. Therefore, it is extremely important to study the genetic changes in breast cancer cells that metastasize to brain and develop specific targeted therapeutic molecular agents.

2. Channelopathy promote breast cancer metastasis

Cancer research is not only focusing on understanding the possible role of transmembrane-BK_{Ca} channels in cancer development and progression but also on development of BK_{Ca} channel modulator drugs to attenuate cancer growth. Several researchers, including us have shown that brain tumor cells express BK_{Ca} and ATP-sensitive potassium (K_{ATP}) channels that are highly responsive to minute changes in intracellular Ca^{2+} and ATP levels. This allows the brain tumor cells to develop pseudopodia for migration through constricted spaces in the brain parenchyma, as depicted in **Figure 1**. Several articles have described the efficacy of BK_{Ca} channel-inhibiting drugs or molecules in reducing tumors in preclinical mouse tumor models. A recent study has shown the role of intracellular BK_{Ca} channels (mitoBK_{Ca}) in cancer cell biology [9, 10].

2.1 Ion channels in breast cancer metastasis

Even now the metastatic breast cancers are incurable. Extensive research has shown that breast cancer metastasis to other organs, including brain is a complicated process. It is widely believed that breast cancer cells escape the primary site

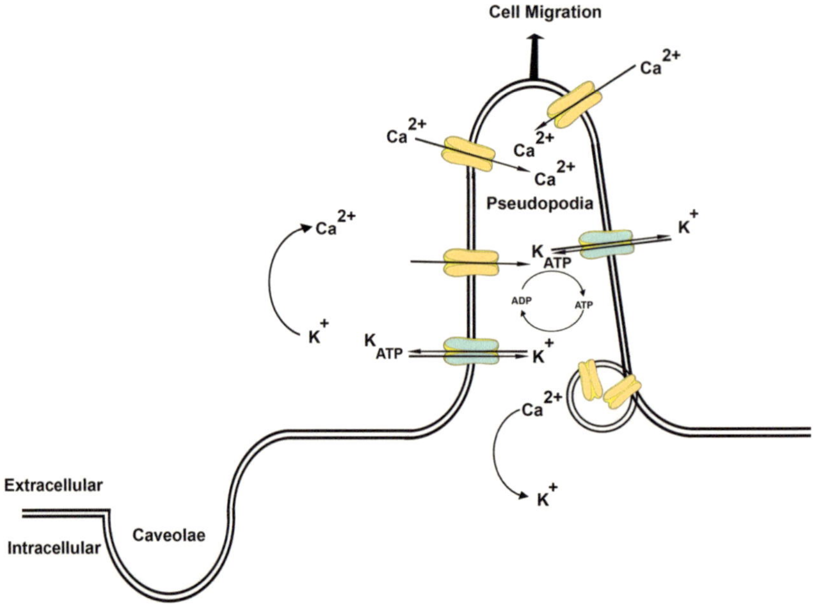

Figure 1.
Anticipated role of BK_{Ca} and K_{ATP} channels in breast cancer cells that seek brain and colonize in brain parenchyma. The potassium ion channels expressed in breast cancer cells are extremely sensitive to minute surge of extracellular and intracellular Ca^{2+} and cause K^+ efflux through BK_{Ca} channels. Similarly, slight imbalance in ADP-ATP levels in the cell causes K^+ efflux through K_{ATP} channels. Then the ion imbalance triggers the Ca^{2+} entry, which promotes cancer cell migration though pseudopodia.

and migrate by lymphatic route to lymph nodes and vascular route to colonize in other organs including brain [11, 12]. Gene-expression profiling studies of breast cancer cells indicate that specific molecular pathways are associated with dissemination of primary tumor cells through a vascular route and not by lymphatic dissemination [12]. There is much interest in studying how and when the cancer cells initiate the metastatic cascade so that a therapeutic intervention can be developed to stop or delay the metastasis. Some cancer researchers [13] believe that targeted treatment of breast cancer with ER/PR modulators (Aromatase inhibitors) and targeted biologics such as Herceptin (Her-2 neu inhibitor) [14] and bevacizumab [15] (anti-vascular). Others argue that the metastasis of cancer cells is triggered by a dysregulated cellular Ca^{2+} homeostasis and altered Ca^{2+} signaling caused by imbalanced fluxes through ion channels and transporters [10, 16]. The BK_{Ca} channels are more sensitive to Ca^{2+} ions in cancer cells. In this regard, we studied whether the increased sensitivity of potentially new BK_{Ca} channel variant protein encoded by splice variants (**Figure 2**) *KCNMA1ΔE2* and *KCNMA1vE22* to intra and extra cellular Ca^{2+} in breast cancer [17]. In fact, a recent evidence indicates that KCa-Ca^{2+} channel complexes were found in cancer cells and contribute to cancer-associated functions such as cell proliferation, cell migration and the capacity to develop metastases [10]. The BK_{Ca} channels are unique since its activity is triggered by depolarization and enhanced by an increase in μM range of intracellular calcium [Ca^{2+}_i]. In this regard, we recently showed that BK_{Ca} channel variant encoded by a new splice variant *KCNMA1vE22* is highly sensitive to [Ca^{2+}_i] and causes glioma progression to high grade glioblastoma multiforme (GBM) [18]. We also discovered a new splice variant *KCNMA1vE22* in breast cancer cells that contributes to breast cancer metastasis to brain (to be published). Epigenetics play an important role in cancer initiation, growth and progression. Understanding the precise mechanism helps us in developing diagnosis, prognosis and treatment strategies for affected cancer patients. For example, overexpression of Ezh2 plays a role in many cancers,

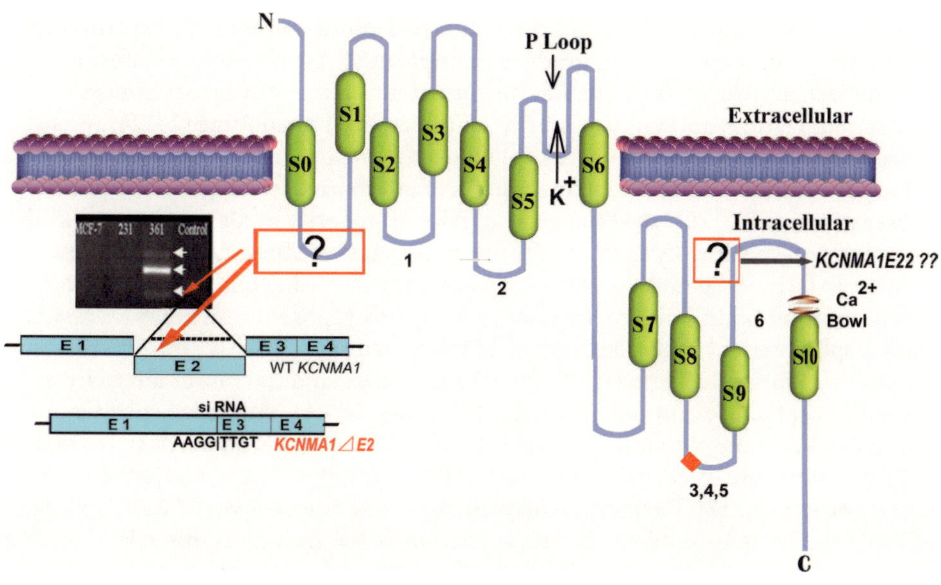

Figure 2.
BK_{Ca} channel is a 7-transmembrane tetramer of four monomeric pore-forming alpha-subunits encoded by KCNMA1. The cytoplasmic C-terminal domain has RCK1 and RCK2 (with calcium bowl) segments. We identified KCNMA1ΔE2 and KCNMA1E22 in human brain-specific metastatic breast cancer cells. Using relevant siRNA designs, we showed that these splice variants are formed by the deletion of exon 2 (E2) and 108 base pair deletion in exon 22 (E22), respectively.

including breast cancer and brain tumors. H3K27M serves as an oncohistone and, if mutated it contributes to tumor development as Ezh2 is no longer able to methylate the histone and gene expression is aberrantly upregulated.

Furthermore, a recent computational analysis of human genomic sequence identified mutations that cause pathogenic splicing abnormalities in breast cancer susceptibility genes, BRCA1, BRCA2 and other genes [19]. Several investigations have reported that voltage gated ion channels are expressed in several cancers and contribute significantly to cell signaling, cell cycle progression and cell volume regulation, cancer cell proliferation, as well as metastasis. Hence, there is a great deal of interest in possible therapeutic potential of voltage gated ion channels as pharmacological targets [20, 21].

2.2 Metastatic breast cancer in brain microenvironment

Cancer cells have the innate ability to "exploit" the "chaotic" environmental challenges surrounding them and grow uninterrupted by manipulating transportome that regulate proliferation, apoptosis, metabolism, growth factor signaling, migration and invasion. Ion channels and transporters are some of the key modulators of cancer progression in hostile tumor microenvironment that includes hypoxia. It has been suggested that modulation of ion channels by the hypoxic environment may contribute to the aggressive phenotype observed in GBM cells residing in a hypoxic environment [22]. In hostile microenvironment such as hypoxia, BK_{Ca} channels are modulated to aid cancer cell invasion and neovascularization. Affymetrix Array analyses of brain tumor cell lines where KCNMA1 was either overexpressed or suppressed showed significant changes in genes involved in cell proliferation, angiogenesis, cell cycle, and invasion [18].

2.3 *KCNMA1*/BK_{Ca} channel splice variants in breast cancer

During the past decade, a number of genes associated with breast cancer have been cloned and identified. Gene expression levels alone cannot fully explain gene function as alternative splicing produce multiple mRNAs and protein isoforms. New molecular insights indicate that the metastatic capacity of breast tumors is an inherent feature, and not necessarily a late, acquired phenotype [23, 24]. Breast cancer cells show alternative mRNA splicing and have prognostic and therapeutic value [21]. Although there are many reports of alternative splicing events specific to breast cancer [25, 26], the biological activity of majority of alternatively spliced isoforms, and specifically their contribution to metastatic breast cancer biology, remains to be investigated. As many researchers are focusing on "Understanding and Preventing Brain Tumor Dispersal", we recently reported on a novel *KCNMA1* mRNA splice variant with a deletion of 108 base pairs (KCNMA1v) mostly overexpressed in high-grade gliomas [18]. In order to understand the role of alternative pre-mRNA splicing events of *KCNMA1*/ BK_{Ca} channels, we employed specific inhibitors. We showed that the modulation of *KCNMA1*/BK_{Ca} channels in brain specific metastatic breast cancer cells (MDA-MB361) resulted in attenuation of migration, invasion [11, 17]. Further, we identified a hitherto unknown *KCNMA1* variant *KCNMA1vE22* (to be published) with a deletion of 108 base pairs of nucleotides and deletion of the entire exon-2 (*KCNMA1ΔE2*) expressed only in metastatic breast tumor cells seeking brain (**Figure 2**). However, biological function of *KCNMA1ΔE2* under different tumor microenvironment is yet to be elucidated. The *KCNMA1* splicing effects and the potential role of *KCNMA1ΔE2* as a critical posttranscriptional regulator of BK_{Ca} channel isoform resulting in diversified channel functions merit further investigation.

Cell line	Proliferation (at 72 h)	Invasion	Trans-endothelial migration	Functional activity	Tumor volume at the 5th week
Untransfected	1 ± 0.09	1 ± 0.10	1 ± 0.17	1 ± 0.11	1 ± 0.21
Vector-transfected	0.98 ± 0.04	1.01 ± 0.12	0.95 ± 0.13	1.2 ± 0.15	1 ± 0.27
KCNMA1vE22-transfected	1.4 ± 0.12	1.9 ± 0.15	1.5 ± 0.19	1.6 ± 0.21	3.8 ± 0.42

Data shown are in SEM of n = 3 in triplicates. Biological function assays [11] and functional activity of BK_{Ca} channels were measured by membrane potential assay using FlexStation and in vivo mouse brain tumor models as described by us earlier.

Table 1.
Effect of KCNMA1vE22 expression on biological functions of MDA-MB-231BR cell line.

Identifying the most optimal and novel biomarker(s) for breast cancer metastasis to brain is ideal [27, 28] yet challenging because of the multi-factorial nature of the disease. The roles of roles of different ion channels in the development of cancer have been reported [29]. The identification of a potential new biomarker has relied heavily on an increase or decrease in gene expression, but these changes may not always result in altered protein expression. Growing evidence indicates that alternative or aberrant pre-mRNA splicing resulting in protein isoforms with diverse functions occurs during the development, progression, and metastasis of breast cancer [29]. Earlier, we have reported that the BK_{Ca} channels play a role in human breast tumor progression, cell proliferation, invasion, and micro-metastases [11, 17]. Nevertheless, the precise role of *KCNMA1* and its splice variants in modification of BK_{Ca} channel functions in promoting breast cancer metastasis to brain is still unclear. Therefore, to understand the role of BK_{Ca} channels in breast cancer metastasis to brain the we showed that the relative messenger RNA levels in MDA-MB-361 cells derived from human metastatic breast tumor in brain were higher than metastatic breast cancer cells (MDA-MB-231) that prefer other organs and primary breast cancer (MCF-7) cells. In addition, using GeneChip Exon array (Affymetrix) we probed the presence of alternative splicing of *KCNMA1* in MDA-MB-361, MDA-MB-231 and MCF-7. The array data showed that *KCNMA1* splicing pattern is different among cell lines with three different phenotypes (to be published).

The PCR results validated the findings of Exon array study. Two distinct splice variants expressed in breast cell line (MDA-MB-361) metastatic to brain were identified (i) deletion of exon 2 (*KCNMA1ΔE2*) between S0-S1 protein subunit (**Figure 2**) corresponding to the cytoplasmic potential domain of BK_{Ca} channel α-subunit and (ii) deletion of 108 bp in exon 22 (*KCNMA1vE22*) between the S9 and S10 protein subunit (C-terminus). However, the biological function of these alternative splice variants in breast cancer remains to be investigated. To our knowledge we believe that our laboratory is the first to report the presence of these variants in metastatic breast cancers. We established that *KCNMA1vE22* plays a key role in several biological functions of MDA-MB-231BR cell line as represented in **Table 1**.

3. BK_{Ca} channels and neovascularization

Altered ion channels could play a pivotal role in physiological angiogenesis in including cancer [30, 31]. BK_{Ca} channel inhibitor modulated the tumorigenic ability of hormone-independent breast cancer cells via the Wnt pathway [32].

Our work shows an association between the BK_{Ca} channel isoform expression and VEGF secretion by breast tumor cells, which might be exacerbated under hypoxia that has implications for vascular permeability and anticancer drug delivery (to be published). Understanding the underlying mechanism and splicing patterns of *KCNMA1* and expression of the splice variant *KCNMA1ΔE2* under normoxia and hypoxia alone and in coculture with brain endothelial cells will shed light on the role of *KCNMA1* alternative splicing in metastatic breast tumor biology. Perhaps the discovery and validation of brain specific metastasis-associated *KCNMA1* alternate splice variants will serve as new tools for the diagnosis and classification of breast tumor patients with high risk of brain metastasis. In fact, splice variations in a number of genes have already been shown to correlate with malignancy and their occurrence could precede clinical cancer diagnosis [33]. To date, however brain-specific alternate *KCNMA1* splice variants in breast cancer have not been reported. The variant *KCNMA1ΔE2* that we have discovered potentially may fill the gap to serve as a biomarker of breast cancer metastasis to brain. Undoubtedly, the research on the putative association between *KCNMA1* splice variants and breast cancer metastases to brain will prove to be an extremely productive exercise for the identification of a new generation of biomarkers. *KCNAM1*/BK_{Ca} channels are hypothesized to be involved in VEGF secretion and neovascularization in brain tumors. We tested this hypothesis by activation and suppression of *KCNMA1* in brain tumor cells and constructed a potential VEGF signaling pathway adapted from KEGG VEGF signaling pathway (**Figure 3**).

We rationalize that *KCNMA1ΔE2* is expressed specifically in metastatic breast tumors in brain, and this requires validation to confirm its role as a potential transformation biomarker of breast cancer metastasis to brain. In metastatic breast tumor cells seeking brain there is an upregulation and constitutive activation of *KCNMA1*, which correlates with increased malignancy [11]. In this context,

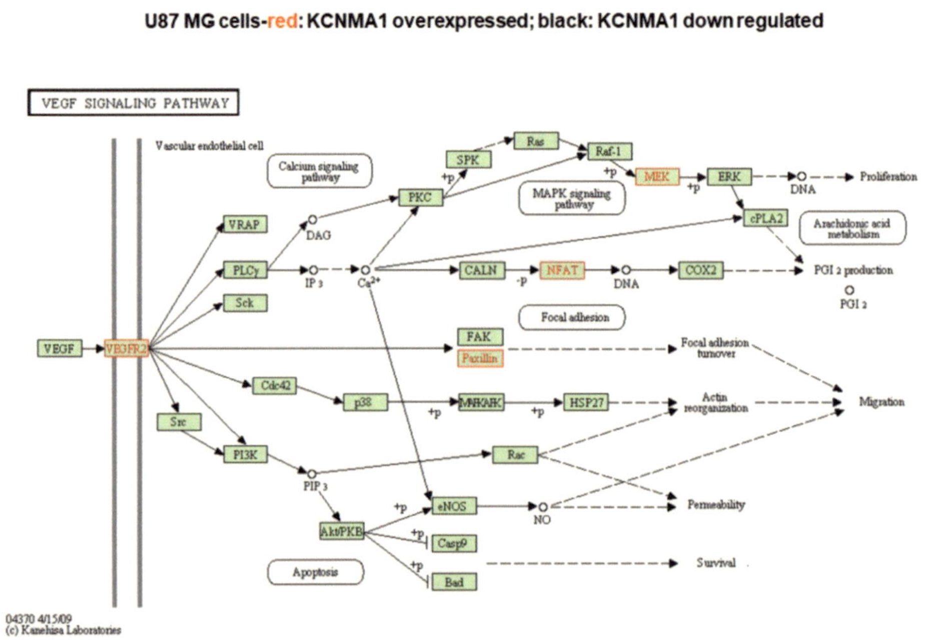

Figure 3.
Adapted from KEGG-VEGF signaling pathway: we activated and suppressed KCNMA1 in brain tumor cells and constructed a probable VEGF signaling pathway affected by modified KCNAMA1 expression. The genes in rectangular boxes—red represents genes overexpressed by KCNMA1 overexpression and black represents genes downregulated by KCNMA1 inhibition in U-87 (glioma cells).

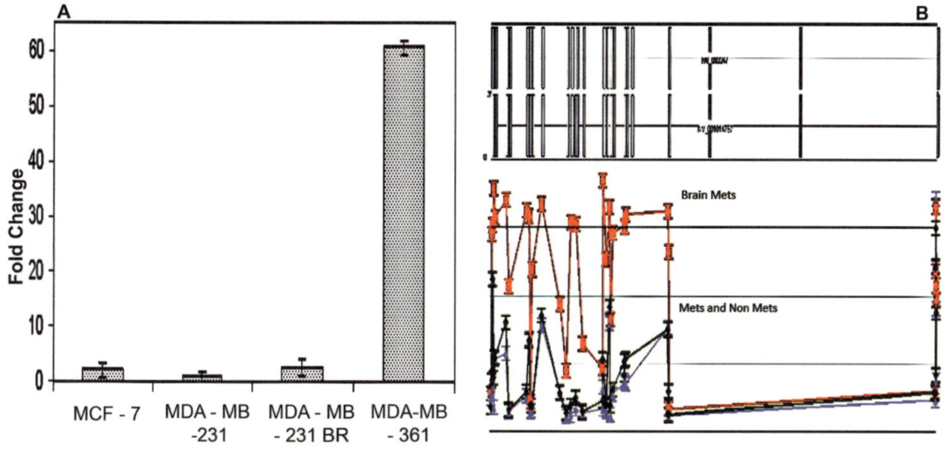

Figure 4.
BK_{Ca} channels in breast cancer biology-expression of KCNMA1 by qPCR (A) and alternate splice variants (B) using Affymetrix Genechip Exon Array in MCF-7 (non Mets), MDA-MB-231 (Mets) and MDA-MB-361 (brain Mets) cell lines.

we showed (**Figure 4**) that the *KCNMA1* is overexpressed in breast cancer cells metastatic to brain (MDA-MB-361) and exhibit differences in expression levels in other non-metastatic (MCF-7) and metastatic to other organs (MDA-MB-231). MDA-MB-231 BR was established from the triple negative MDA-MB-231 cells, which are highly metastatic but have no organ specificity. The MDA-MB 231-BR cell line was derived from MDA-MB-231 cells following sequential rounds of implantation, resection from the brain, and re-injection into mice. Eventually a subline with selectivity for the brain was isolated [34], and exhibit higher KCNMA1 level than parental MDA-MB-231 cells, however the expression was far lower than the naturally-selected MDA-MB-361 cells (**Figure 4**).

In addition, alternate splicing of *KCNMA1* [17] including *KCNMA1ΔE2* may provide a mechanism to generate a physiologically diverse complement of functionally and structurally diverse BK_{Ca} channel isoform that might affect cell proliferation, cell cycle, migration and micrometastases in brain. Future studies will validate the role of *KCNMA1ΔE2* in brain-specific metastatic process. Inhibiting *KCNMA1ΔE2 in in vitro* and *in vivo* models with shRNA or the variant BK_{Ca} channel using specific inhibitor like Iberiotoxin to attenuate breast tumor metastasis to brain using human metastatic breast tumor xenograft mouse models will be very stimulating.

4. Discussion

4.1 Splicing in health and disease

Many human diseases are implicated to errors in mRNA splicing. These aberrant splicing also provides an opportunity to develop targeted treatment to correct the faulty gene in some genetic disorders, or target aberrant protein encoded by these gene variants in human cancers. Breast cancer-specific biomarkers might generate specific epitopes that offer targets for developing diagnostic, prognostic and immunotherapy [35]. Articles on alternative pre-mRNA splicing regulation in cancer [36] and misregulation of mRNA splicing in cancer [29] highlights the important roles in promoting aberrant splicing, which in turn contributes to all aspects of tumor biology.

4.2 BK_{Ca} channels as target to attenuate breast cancer metastasis

The BK_{Ca} channels are known to function as oncogenes in certain cancers. These channels besides being sensitive to $[Ca^{2+}{}_i]$ are highly dependent on amounts of outward K^+ currents, which modulate the transmembrane potential of a cell. The BK_{Ca} channels are overexpressed in many types of cancers via gene amplification, alternative splicing or increased protein half-life. A recent study showed that by inhibiting BK_{Ca} channels with Iberiotoxin in breast cancer cells, tumorigenicity was reduced by downregulation of β-catenin and (phospho)Akt and HER-2/neu protein levels [37]. Evidence presented above clearly show that over expression of wild type BK_{Ca} channels or the presence of BK_{Ca} channel variant support breast cancer metastasis to brain. Understanding the mechanism of its action in brain metastasis will provide a unique opportunity to identify and differentiate between low grade breast cancers that are at high risk for metastasis from those at low risk for metastasis. This distinction would in turn allow for the appropriate and efficient application of effective diagnosis, prognosis and treatments while sparing patients with low risk for metastasis from the toxic side effects of chemotherapy. Activation of BK_{Ca} channels was shown to be a novel molecular pathway involved in zoledronic acid-induced apoptosis of MDA-MB-231 cells *in vitro* [32]. Du et al. [8] showed that BK_{Ca} promotes growth and metastasis of prostate cancer through facilitating the coupling between αvβ3 integrin and FAK. BK_{Ca} channels are shown to support cancer cell migration, invasion and tumorigenesis [11, 17, 18]. Hence it is extremely interesting to explore BK_{Ca} channels as putative targets for anti-breast cancer therapies.

4.3 Alternate splicing of BK_{Ca} channels in diagnosis and prognosis

Several articles have highlighted the use of alternative splicing as a promising source for new diagnostic, prognostic, predictive, and therapeutic tools [38–40]. The diversity of RNA species detected through RNA-seq holds the potential of extracellular RNAs as non-invasive diagnostic indicators of disease [41–44]. We recently reported that targeting the KCNMA1 variants may be a clinically beneficial strategy to prevent or at least slow down glioma transformation to GBM [18]. In both human and mouse lymphoma models, researchers have shown that MYC directly induced the transcription of genes encoding core splicing machinery components. They also showed that PRMT5 is involved in MYC-driven tumorigenesis in mice with lymphoma and discovered that tumor development was delayed [44]. Now due to high-throughput New Generation Sequencing (NGS) technologies the splicing diagnostic methodologies have improved. Hence NGS can be utilized in clinical diagnostics of splice variants in diagnosis, prognosis and treatment of breast cancers.

4.4 Perspective of *KCNMA1* splice variants

We believe that future therapies for metastatic breast cancer depend on further investigation into the mechanisms and cellular events caused by oncogene splicing such as *KCNMA1*. Such studies should lead to the development of future therapies for this deadly type of cancer. *KCNMA1* splice variants that are identified in breast tumor patients with brain metastasis will pave for accurate diagnosis and prognostication. Furthermore, they provide potential targets for anticancer drug development. Clinical outcome of *KCNMA1vE22* expression in breast metastasis is expected to reveal the variants' clinical importance. Quantifying the levels of *KCNMA1vE22* could be useful to identify biological process that increases the malignancy and affect prognosis of patients with breast cancer metastasis in the brain.

5. Conclusions

Perhaps the discovery and validation of brain specific metastasis-associated *KCNMA1* alternate splice variants will serve as new tools for the diagnosis and classification of breast tumor patients with high risk of brain metastasis. In fact, splice variations in a number of genes have already been shown to correlate with malignancy and their occurrence could precede clinical cancer diagnosis. To date, however brain-specific alternate *KCNMA1* splice variants in breast cancer have not been reported. The variant *KCNMA1ΔE2* and *KCNMA1E22* that we have recently discovered potentially may fill the gap to serve as a biomarker of breast cancer metastasis to brain. Undoubtedly, the research on the putative association between *KCNMA1* splice variants and breast cancer metastases to brain will prove to be an extremely productive research to identify new generation of biomarkers for early detection and therapeutic intervention in breast cancer patients with high risk for brain metastases.

Acknowledgements

The authors thank the Scintilla Group, Bangalore, India; Anderson Cancer Institute and Mercer University Medical Center, Savannah, GA, USA; Vanderbilt-Ingram Cancer Center, Nashville, TN, USA; Cedars-Sinai Medical Center, Los Angeles, CA, USA; American Cancer Society, USA; Georgia Cancer Coalition, Atlanta, GA, USA; and NIH for providing opportunity and research grant support. We also thank Dr. Nagendra of MVIT, Bangalore, for assisting us with the STRING software for the analysis and Michigan State University Research Center, Grand Rapids, MI, USA, for generating KKEG pathway using Affymetrix analysis data.

Author details

Divya Khaitan[1] and Nagendra Ningaraj[1,2]*

1 Department of Molecular Oncology, Scintilla Academy for Applied Sciences' Education and Research, Bangalore, India

2 Molecular Diagnostics Labs, Scintilla Bio-MARC, Bangalore, India

*Address all correspondence to: sainagendra50@gmail.com

References

[1] Tosoni A, Franceschi E, Brandes AA. Chemotherapy in breast cancer patients with brain metastases: Have new chemotherapic agents changed the clinical outcome? Critical Reviews in Oncology/Hematology. 2008;**68**:212-221. DOI: 10.1016/j.critrevonc.2008.04.004

[2] Lin NU, Carey LA, Liu MC, Younger J, Come SE, Ewend M, et al. Phase II Trial of lapatinib for brain metastases in patients with human epidermal growth factor receptor 2-positive breast cancer. Journal of Clinical Oncology: Official Journal of the American Society of Clinical Oncology. 2008;**26**(12):1993. DOI: 10.1200/JCO.2007.12.3588

[3] Boogerd W, Vos VW, Hart AA, Baris G. Brain metastases in breast cancer; natural history, prognostic factors and outcome. Journal of Neuro-oncology. 1993;**15**(2):165-174. DOI: 10.1007/BF01053937

[4] Distefano A, Yap HY, Hortobagyi GN, Blumenschein GR. The natural history of breast cancer patients with brain metastases. Cancer. 1979;**44**(5):1913-1918. DOI: 10.1002/1097-0142(197911)44:5<1913::AID-CNCR2820440554>3.0.CO;2-D

[5] Sparrow GE, Rubens RD. Brain metastases from breast cancer: Clinical course, prognosis and influence of treatment. Clinical Oncology. 1981;**7**(4):291

[6] Bos PD, Zhang XH, Nadal C, Shu W, Gomis RR, Nguyen DX, et al. Genes that mediate breast cancer metastasis to the brain. Nature. 2009;**459**(7249):100

[7] Klein A, Olendrowitz C, Schmutzler R, Hampl J, Schlag PM, Maass N, et al. Identification of brain-and bone-specific breast cancer metastasis genes. Cancer Letters. 2009;**276**(2):212-220. DOI: 10.1016.2008.11.017

[8] Du C, Zheng Z, Li D, Chen L, Li N, Yi X, et al. BKCa promotes growth and metastasis of prostate cancer through facilitating the coupling between αvβ3 integrin and FAK. Oncotarget. 2016;**7**(26):40174. DOI: 10.18632/oncotarget.9559

[9] Rao V, Perez-Neut M, Kaja S, Gentile S. Voltage-gated ion channels in cancer cell proliferation. Cancers. 2015;**7**(2):849-875. DOI: 10.3390/cancers7020813

[10] Gueguinou M, Chantome A, Fromont G, Bougnoux P, Vandier C, Potier-Cartereau M. KCa and Ca^{2+} channels: The complex thought. Biochimica et Biophysica Acta (BBA)-Molecular Cell Research. 2014;**1843**(10):2322-2333. DOI: 10.1016/j.bbamcr.2014.02.019

[11] Khaitan D, Sankpal UT, Weksler B, Meister EA, Romero IA, Couraud PO, et al. Role of KCNMA1 gene in breast cancer invasion and metastasis to brain. BMC Cancer. 2009;**9**(1):258. DOI: 10.1186/1471-2407-9-258

[12] Pantel K, Brakenhoff RH. Dissecting the metastatic cascade. Nature Reviews Cancer. 2004;**4**(6):448-456. DOI: 10.1038/nrc1370

[13] Kümler I, Knoop AS, Jessing CA, Ejlertsen B, Nielsen DL. Review of hormone-based treatments in postmenopausal patients with advanced breast cancer focusing on aromatase inhibitors and fulvestrant. ESMO Open. 2016;**1**(4):e000062. DOI: 10.1136/esmoopen-2016-000062

[14] Maximiano S, Magalhaes P, Guerreiro MP, Morgado M. Trastuzumab in the treatment of breast cancer.

BioDrugs. 2016;**30**(2):75-86. DOI: 10.1007/s4025

[15] Kümler I, Christiansen OG, Nielsen DL. A systematic review of bevacizumab efficacy in breast cancer. Cancer Treatment Reviews. 2014;**40**(8):960-973. DOI: 10.1016.2014.05.006

[16] Cui C, Merritt R, Fu L, Pan Z. Targeting calcium signaling in cancer therapy. Actapharmaceuticasinica B. 2017;**7**(1):3-17. DOI: 10.1016.2016.11.001

[17] Khaitan D, Sankpal U, Ningaraj N. An alternative splice variant of KCNMA1 drives breast cancer metastasis and invasion. Cancer Research. 2009;**69**(24 Supplement): 6166. DOI: 10.1158/0008-5472. SABCS-09-6166

[18] Khaitan D, Ningaraj N, Joshua LB. Role of an alternatively spliced KCNMA1 variant in glioma growth. In: Brain Tumors—An Update. Rijeka: IntechOpen; 2018. DOI: 10.5772/ INTECHOPEN.74509

[19] Apostolou P, Fostira F. Hereditary breast cancer: The era of new susceptibility genes. BioMed Research International. 2013;**2013**. DOI: 10.1155/2013/747318

[20] Weigelt B, Peterse JL, Van't Veer LJ. Breast cancer metastasis: Markers and models. Nature Reviews Cancer. 2005;**5**(8):591. DOI: 10.1038/ nrc1670

[21] Martínez-Montiel N, Anaya-Ruiz M, Pérez-Santos M, Martínez-Contreras R. Alternative splicing in breast cancer and the potential development of therapeutic tools. Genes. 2017;**8**(10):217. DOI: 10.3390/ genes8100217

[22] Peruzzo R, Biasutto L, Szabò I, Leanza L. Impact of intracellular ion channels on cancer development and progression. European Biophysics Journal. 2016;**45**(7):685-707. DOI: 10.1007/s00249-016-1143-0

[23] Sforna L, Cenciarini M, Belia S, D'Adamo MC, Pessia M, Franciolini F, et al. The role of ion channels in the hypoxia-induced aggressiveness of glioblastoma. Frontiers in Cellular Neuroscience. 2015;**15**(8):467. DOI: 10.3389/fncel.2014.00467

[24] Wang W, Eddy R, Condeelis J. The cofilin pathway in breast cancer invasion and metastasis. Nature Reviews Cancer. 2007;**7**(6):429. DOI: 10.1038/nrc2148

[25] Wang ET, Sandberg R, Luo S, Khrebtukova I, Zhang L, Mayr C, et al. Alternative isoform regulation in human tissue transcriptomes. Nature. 2008;**456**(7221):470. DOI: 10.1038/ nature07509

[26] Venables JP, Klinck R, Bramard A, Inkel L, Dufresne-Martin G, Koh C, et al. Identification of alternative splicing markers for breast cancer. Cancer Research. 2008;**68**(22):9525-9531. DOI: 10.1158/0008-5472. CAN-08-1769

[27] Li J, Zhang N, Song LB, Liao WT, Jiang LL, Gong LY, et al. Astrocyte elevated gene-1 is a novel prognostic marker for breast cancer progression and overall patient survival. Clinical Cancer Research. 2008;**14**(11):3319-3326. DOI: 10.1158/1078-0432. CCR-07-4054

[28] Roy R, Yang J, Moses MA. Matrix metalloproteinases as novel biomarkers and potential therapeutic targets in human cancer. Journal of Clinfical Oncology. 2009;**27**(31):5287. DOI: 10.1200/JCO.2009.23.5556

[29] David CJ, Manley JL. Alternative pre-mRNA splicing regulation in cancer: Pathways and programs unhinged. Genes & Development.

2010;**24**(21):2343-2364. DOI: 10.1101/gad.1973010

[30] Li M, Xiong ZG. Ion channels as targets for cancer therapy. International Journal of Physiology, Pathophysiology and Pharmacology. 2011;**3**(2):156

[31] Munaron L, Genova T, Avanzato D, Antoniotti S, Fiorio Pla A. Targeting calcium channels to block tumor vascularization. Recent Patents on Anti-cancer Drug Discovery. 2013;**8**(1):27-37. DOI: 10.2174/15748921380390212 5

[32] Schickling BM, England SK, Aykin-Burns N, Norian LA, Leslie KK, Frieden-Korovkina VP. BKCa channel inhibitor modulates the tumorigenic ability of hormone-independent breast cancer cells via the Wnt pathway. Oncology Reports. 2015;**33**(2):533-538. DOI: 10.3892/OR.2014.3617

[33] Srivastava S, Grizzle WE. Biomarkers and the genetics of early neoplastic lesions. Cancer Biomarkers. 2011;**9**(1-6):41-64. DOI: 10.3233/CBM-2011-0204

[34] Yoneda T, Williams PJ, Hiraga T, Niewolna M, Nishimura R. A bone-seeking clone exhibits different biological properties from the MDA-MB-231 parental human breast cancer cells and a brain-seeking clone in vivo and in vitro. Journal of Bone and Mineral Research. 2001;**16**:1486-1495. DOI: 10.1359/jbmr.2001.16.8.1486

[35] Douglas AG, Wood MJ. RNA splicing: Disease and therapy. Briefings in functional genomics. 2011;**10**(3):151-164. DOI: 10.1093/bfgp/elr020

[36] Kalniņa Z, Zayakin P, Siliņa K, Linē A. Alterations of pre-mRNA splicing in cancer. Genes, Chromosomes and Cancer. 2005;**42**(4):342-357. DOI: 10.1002/gcc.20156

[37] Zhang J, Manley JL. Misregulation of pre-mRNA alternative splicing in cancer. Cancer Discovery. 2013;**3**(11):1228-1237. DOI: 10.1158/2159-8290.CD-13-0253

[38] Bezzi M, Teo SX, Muller J, Mok WC, Sahu SK, Vardy LA, et al. Regulation of constitutive and alternative splicing by PRMT5 reveals a role for Mdm4 pre-mRNA in sensing defects in the spliceosomal machinery. Genes & Development. 2013;**27**(17):1903-1916. DOI: 10.1101/gad.219899.113

[39] Ma YG, Liu WC, Dong S, Du C, Wang XJ, Li JS, et al. Activation of BKCa channels in zoledronic acid-induced apoptosis of MDA-MB-231 breast cancer cells. PLoS One. 2012;**7**(5):e37451. DOI: 10.1371/journal.pone.0037451

[40] Baralle D, Buratti E. RNA splicing in human disease and in the clinic. Clinical Science. 2017;**131**(5):355-368. DOI: 10.1042/CS20160211

[41] Pajares MJ, Ezponda T, Catena R, Calvo A, Pio R, Montuenga LM. Alternative splicing: An emerging topic in molecular and clinical oncology. The Lancet Oncology. 2007;**8**(4):349-357. DOI: 10.1016/S1470-2045(07)70104-3

[42] Klinck R, Bramard A, Inkel L, Dufresne-Martin G, Gervais-Bird J, Madden R, et al. Multiple alternative splicing markers for ovarian cancer. Cancer Research. 2008;**68**(3):657-663. DOI: 10.1158/0008-5472.CAN-07-2580

[43] Anczuków O, Akerman M, Cléry A, Wu J, Shen C, Shirole NH, et al. SRSF1-regulated alternative splicing in breast cancer. Molecular Cell. 2015;**60**(1):105-117. DOI: 10.1016/j.molcel.2015.09.005

[44] Byron SA, Van Keuren-Jensen KR, Engelthaler DM, Carpten JD, Craig DW. Translating RNA sequencing into clinical diagnostics: Opportunities and challenges. Nature Reviews Genetics. 2016;**17**(5):257. DOI: 10.1038/nrg.2016.10

Section 3

Different Treatment Strategies for Breast Cancer

Chapter 5

Targeted Breast Cancer Treatment Using New Photochemotherapeutic Compounds

Ivan Sosthene Mfouo Tynga and Heidi Abrahamse

Abstract

The deregulation of cell growth in milk-producing glands, milk-carrying tubes, or connective tissues is known as breast cancer. It originates from genetic mutations and has the ability to metastasize. Primary tumor cells repetitively divide and lead to inappropriate mechanisms, tumorigenesis, and carcinogenesis, characterized by improper cell type, function, lifetime, and self-destruction. The tumor-specific activation is considered to be an effective strategy for selective cancer destruction, which remains an issue with conventional therapeutic approaches. The tumor microenvironment can be regulated and adapted through an interaction between pH, proteins, and other factors. Principally, human breast cancer genes, BRCA1 and BRCA2, produce tumor suppressors that prevent changes in genetic materials, as well as ensure their stability. Photodynamic therapy is a targeted cancer modality that depends on the photochemotherapeutic agent and light characteristics used to activate the compound. The possibility of eradicating breast cancer depends on continuous development of therapeutic approaches using third-generation photochemotherapeutic compounds to improve targeting this cancer and its stem cells.

Keywords: breast cancer, cell cycle regulation, genetic mutation, tumor microenvironment, cancer therapies, new photosensitizers

1. Introduction

Both males and females have breasts, which are composed of adipose (fat) tissues, supplied by nerves, blood vessels, lymph nodes and vessels, connective tissues, and ligaments. The breasts superimpose the pectoral muscles and are predominantly pronounced in females after puberty. Breasts consist of mammary glands that contain at least a dozen of lobes, further subdivided into lobules, and stimulated lobules are able to initiate and produce milk. The lobules are specially structured and connected to a system of ductal channels to deliver milk to the nipple. The glandular and ductal structures are surrounded by dense fat and connective tissues, which determine the size of a breast (**Figure 1**) [1, 2]. This anatomy is completed by a network of connective tissues, ligaments, nerves, and both lymph and blood vessels for proper structural and functional processing [3].

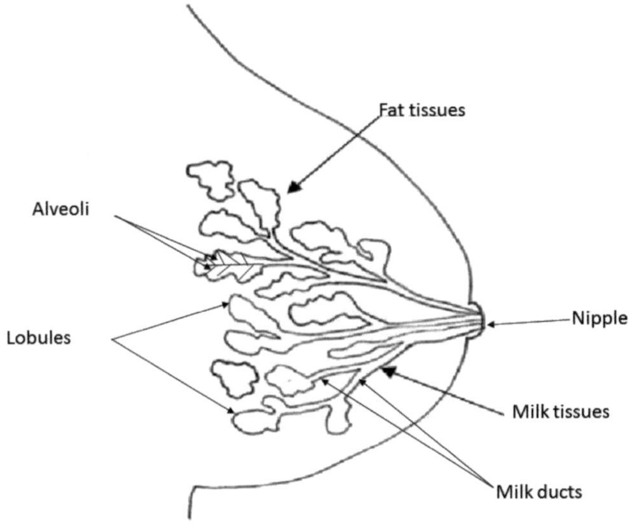

Figure 1.
Schematic representation of the breast. Milk passages from the alveoli through the milk ducts to the nipple during breast feeding.

Like any other cell cycle, the breast cell cycle endures proper cell proliferation and functioning by duplicating cell genetic materials and giving off two daughter cells during each cycle. It consists of four distinctive phases and in the first or quiescence phase (G0), the cell remains in a resting state, where cell division is stationary. The second is known as the intermitotic phase and is further subdivided into a gap 1 phase (a prior-DNA synthesis stage) in which cell size increase and control mechanisms ensure readiness for DNA replication (genetic synthesis) and post-DNA synthesis (gap 2) to ensure readiness for actual cell division. The mitotic phase or sequential cell division consists of prophase, metaphase, anaphase, and telophase. The fourth and final is the cytokinesis phase in which the cytoplasm of eukaryotic cells is divided into two identical cells [4, 5]. To guarantee the integrity of this outcome, a special group of cyclin-dependent kinases (CDKs) play crucial roles in regulating cell cycle progression and are also involved in other processes including regulation of transcription, mRNA processing, and differentiation [6, 7]. When combined with cyclins in dividing cells, stimulated CDKs regulate the sequential events of cell cycle and ensure proper cell division [6]. Cyclins belong to a family of proteins without catalytic ability, expressed at specific subcellular locations, but are able to bind to CDKs and activate the regulatory and catalytic activities [8]. The regulation of downstream proteins and specific cell cycle checkpoints at different phases of cell cycle is dictated by the cyclin-CDK interactions and combinations of those. For instance, during the G1 phase, the combination of cyclin D-CDK4 and cyclin E-CDK2 induces phosphorylation of Rb protein, subsequent activation of E2F proteins, and further expression of E2F reactive genes. These genes encode for cell cycle regulators responsible for G1/S transition. Similarly, during G2 phase, the combination of cyclin A-CDK2 and cyclin B-CDK1 prompts phosphorylation and activation of FoxM1 and recruitment of a histone deacetylase p300/Creb-binding protein that further leads to the expression of FoxM1 target genes. These genes encode for cell cycle regulators that are essential for the mitosis and effectors of the chromosomal segregation (**Figure 2**) [9].

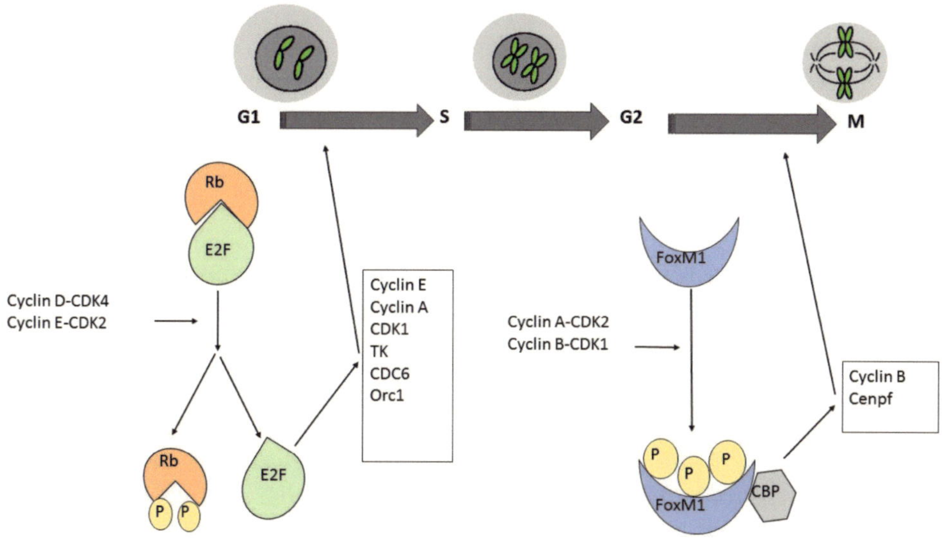

Figure 2.
Cyclin-dependent kinase (CDK) combinations control Rb/E2F- and FoxM1-induced transcription. During the G1 phase, cyclin D-CDK4 and cyclin E-CDK2 combinations disassemble Rb-E2F dimer and phosphorylate Rb, causing the activation of E2F proteins and the expression of E2F-responsive genes. The genes encode for cell cycle regulators required for G1/S transition (cyclin E, cyclin A, CDK1, TK, CDC6, and Orc1). During the G2 phase, cyclin A-CDK2 and cyclin B-CDK1 combinations phosphorylate and activate FoxM1, causing the recruitment of a histone deacetylase p300/CBP that further activates the expression of FoxM1 target genes. These genes encode for mitotic regulators (cyclin B) and chromosomal segregation effectors (Cenpf). Rb = retinoblastoma protein CDK = cyclin-dependent kinase, TK = thymidine kinase, CDC6 = components of the DNA replication machinery, Orc1 = origin recognition complex subunit 1, CBP = CREB binding protein, Cenpf = centromere protein factor.

2. Genetic mutation and types of breast cancer

Abnormal expression or change occurring in the activity of cyclin-CDK combinations leads to the loss of cell cycle control, where cells no longer follow the distinctive progression and go into a malignant formation [6]. Breast cancer is a heterogeneous disease characterized by change in morphology, invasive behavior, metastatic ability, and hormone receptor expression, leading to malignant cells multiplication in breasts with ability to spread to other parts of the body, if the condition is not treated [10, 11]. Breast cancer is the most commonly diagnosed invasive cancer in women, and second main reason of cancer-related death, after lung cancer. Common symptoms include and are not limited to thickness of breast tissues, lumps in the armpits, persistent pain through monthly cycle, pigmentation change or peeling or scaling of the skin of the breast, altered breast size and shape, inverted nipples and rash around the nipple area with a likely discharge [11]. Mutations in some genes controlling checkpoints like the cell cycle inhibitors, Rb and p53 may induce dysregulated cell cycle and so encourage tumor formation [12]. These strategic checkpoints prevent cell cycle progression till the verification of essential phase processes and nuclear repair have been completed. Other genes like BRCA, which is an abbreviation for breast cancer gene, have been found influencing the development of breast cancer. In fact, there are two types of BRCA genes, BRCA 1 and BRCA 2, and they do not cause but prevent breast cancer by repairing DNA breaks, which could encourage uncontrolled growth of tumors and cancer. Thus, BRCA genes are tumor suppressor genes. However, in some people (around 1 in 400), these tumor suppressor genes do not function properly, leading to gene mutation. When mutated, BRCA genes can no longer carry out their function of repairing broken DNA and preventing breast cancer. Due to this genetic malfunction, mutated BRCA gene carriers are more prone to develop breast cancer even at a younger age and can equally pass this mutation down to offspring. This seems to be rare with less than 10% of diagnosed women having BRCA mutation. Individuals with the BRCA1 mutation have 55–65% chance of developing cancer before age 70, compared to a lesser portion, 45%, for individuals with the BRCA2 mutation. The BRCA1 mutation is the worse of the two and BRCA1 mutated individuals are more likely to develop a triple negative breast cancer, a hormone dependent form, more aggressive and lesser curable, with higher risk of developing second cancer after successful treatment, known as breast cancer recurrence. However, the majority of breast cancer cases can be successfully cured when detected early, even those with a BRCA1 or BRCA2 mutation [13].

There are several types of breast cancers, and ductal carcinoma in situ (DCIS) is a non-metastatic and non-invasive type that occurs in the ductal cells and this type might be highly curable. Lobular carcinoma (LCIS) is another in situ non-metastatic and non-invasive type, which occurs in cells of the milk-manufacturing lobules, but has the potential to evolve into an invasive type of breast cancer. The most common type is certainly the invasive ductal carcinoma that occurs in the ductal cells and then invades other breast areas with metastatic abilities. Similarly, the invasive lobular carcinoma starts in the lobules and has metastatic abilities; however, it is a very uncommon type of breast cancer. The breast cyst is a noncancerous (benign) type with fluid-filled sac that may be drained. This type is usually diagnosed in females who are in their 30s or 40s. Another early and noncancerous solid type is breast fibroadenoma, commonly affecting vicenarian and tricenarian women in their 20s and 30s and is characterized by the presence of a pain-free and mobile lump in the breast. Fibrocystic breast is a common noncancerous condition with a breast lump that may be altered throughout the menstrual cycle. The breast hyperplasia is characterized by the abnormal proliferation of noncancerous cells in ductal areas and may increase the risk of developing breast cancer. An atypical breast hyperplasia may develop either in ductal or lobular areas and might significantly increase the rsik of breast cancer by four to five times when compared to a healthy woman. The intraductal papilloma is a noncancerous wart-like growth within the ducts that may cause bloody fluid leakage from the nipple. Another noncancerous condition is breast adenosis that is caused by lobular expansion and has to be diligently diagnosed, as it may resemble breast cancer in some occurrences. Another difficult to diagnose type of breast cancer (as it might bear a resemblance to fibroadenoma) is phyllodes tumor, a rare and immense breast tumor that may be benign or malignant and develop around age 40. Fat necrosis may seem like breast cancer but is a lump scar tissue as a result of repairs occurring in the fat tissues of the breast. Commonly occurring in nursing mothers, mastitis is an inflammation of the breast as a result of infection accompanied by redness, pain, warmth, and swelling. Breast calcification refers to the calcium deposits in the breast and has to be diagnosed accordingly, as it may suggest something else. More and more seen is the overdevelopment of male breasts, known as gynecomastia, and it may affect men of all ages [14, 15].

3. Chemistry, pathophysiology, and staging of breast cancer

The characteristics of the environments where breast cancer develops are similar to those of any other cancer. In order to survive, cancer cells must maintain a suitable acid-base balance. As a result of extensive carbon dioxide and lactic acid production, cancer cells are constantly experiencing acid–base fluxes, which severely affect the pH, especially intracellular pH. To maintain a suitable intracellular pH level, specialized pH-dependent transporters regulate the exchange of H^+ or HCO_3^- ions [16]. These specialized proteins are able to induce pH changes by facilitating new interactions or eliminating others [17]. Cancer cells need substantial input of energy for their ever-increasing metabolic demand. Human tumors tend to grow around blood vessels, causing extracellular acidity in tumors and outermost cells to become necrotic. The low microenvironmental oxygen tension and pH are the hallmarks of cancer [18–20]. Swiftly, tumors become poorly perfused and require extra diffusion mechanisms, and carbonic anhydrase plays essential functions in controlling extracellular pH and giving cancer cells alternatives to adjust to micro-environmental acidity and drive disease progression [16].

Although individuals with family history of breast and ovarian cancers have higher risk, both myoepithelial and epithelial cells found in the stratified epithelium of breast are understood to be able to initiate breast carcinogenesis or stem cells that give rise to them [21, 22]. Immune mechanisms aim to identify and destroy cancer cells and DNA-damaged cells. Moreover, RAS/MEK/ERK and PI3K/AKT pathways control the mechanisms of cell suicidal events. Breast cancer commonly arises due to genetic mutations and environmental factors that alter these mechanisms. Exposure of epithelial and/or stromal cells to a certain level of estrogen or adipose-derived hormones or signaling factors can promote cell proliferation and carcinogenesis in breast [23, 24]. Telomerases cease to perform chromosomal shortening roles, extensive cell replication occurs, cancer cells continue to proliferate beyond boundaries through blood and lymph systems, and form secondary tumors [25, 26].

The deepness, size, and type determine the stage of breast cancer from non-invasive to metastatic tumor [27]. Starting in confined localization, tumor initiates without evidence in neighboring cells and a well-known instance of stage 0 breast cancer is DCIS [28]. The next is the invasive stage and is characterized by two categories: stage 1A is a tumor with a diameter lesser than 2 cm and absent in lymph nodes, while stage 1B describes a tumor greater than 2 cm in diameter and present in lymph nodes [29]. Then, there are two other sub-categories where 2A designates tumor localization in axillary lymph nodes with a diameter lesser than 5 cm and 2B tumor has a diameter greater than 5 centimeters and is not in axillary lymph nodes [30]. The third stage is characterized by three sub-categories: 3A describes tumor in 4–9 axillary lymph nodes, while 3B tumor can be inflammatory or not with up to 9 axillary lymph nodal sites and is able to cause ulcer and various skin alterations including red, warm, and swollen breast skin. Stage 3C describes a tumor affecting at least 10 axillary lymph nodal sites and area below the clavicle [31]. The final and advanced stage 4 defines a metastatic tumor that has spread to other organs like lungs, bones, liver, brain, and others [32].

4. Some of the current breast cancer therapies and limitations

Breast feeding women have a lesser risk of developing breast cancer and the defensive mechanisms have not yet been identified [33]. Breast cancer treatments differ and depend on the stage, mass, site, metastatic ability or not of the condition, and the health status of the patient. Currently, the main forms of treatment for breast cancer employ surgery, radiation therapy, hormone therapy, and chemotherapeutic agents [15]. Surgery is the foremost utilized strategy for non-metastasized breast cancer and varies according to the affected tissues [34]. Lumpectomy is known as a breast-conserving surgery, where a partial mastectomy procedure is performed at initial stages of the condition and aims to save the major part of the breast by removing the affected breast part, together with limited healthy tissues and surrounding lymph nodes. It is often complemented with other forms of treatment in order to prevent mastectomies [35]. However, some of the adverse effects are removal of healthy tissues along with the cancer, soreness, short-term inflammation, altered breast appearance, and sclerosis [36]. When not the first choice, mastectomy is often recommended whenever the disease persist after lumpectomy was not sufficient. Nevertheless, the loss of breast is usually accompanied with a profound sense of loss of a woman's self-esteem and further depression in most women [37]. Radiation therapy utilizes high-energy rays to eradicate cancer cells and highly proliferating cells, like those in nails, skin hairs, and others as well. Brachytherapy is a faster partial breast irradiation that directs radiation mostly to and around the affected cancer area, which is better than to irradiate the entire breast [38].

Estrogen and progesterone receptors play important roles in the management of breast cancer as they are used to enhance the selectivity of the treatment. Hormone-dependent treatments using estrogen receptors yield better responses than those with progesterone [39]. The anti-estrogen drugs are commonly used for breast cancer treatments. Tamoxifen had been one of the foremost of these drugs and highly recommended for women with positive estrogen receptor breast carcinoma. Tamoxifen prevents estrogen from entering into breast cancer cells and further development of the condition [40]. Although its therapeutic efficacy for breast cancer has relatively low adverse effects when compared to other anti-estrogen counterparts, this anti-estrogen drug tends to compete with estrogen for binding to estrogen receptors in breast and other organs including uterus, liver, and bones [41]. Both raloxifene and tamoxifen are recognized as selective estrogen receptor regulators and able to prevent or stimulate estrogen-like activity in different tissues by disturbing the estrogen receptors [42]. Additionally, various side effects are associated with the use of anti-estrogen agents, and tamoxifen affects venous thrombosis, cataract, endometrial cancer, menstrual disorders, and hot flushes, while raloxifen brought about lesser damages in some cases and minor danger of cataract and thromboembolism than tamoxifen [43, 44]. Chemotherapy can be used prior to surgery or postsurgery depending on the condition of the patient; it refers to the usage of medicines to eradicate rapidly proliferating and metastatic cancer cells or to minimize their development [45]. The most commonly used chemotherapeutic medicines are Docetaxel, Paclitaxel, Cisplatin, Carboplatin, Vinorelbine, Capecitabine, Liposomal doxorubicin, Cyclophosphamide, and Carboplatin, and they are associated with numerous side effects [46, 47].

5. Targeted breast cancer therapy

Sometimes, the success of treatment is hindered by drug resistance, which has emerged as a main concern for the fight against cancer. Targeted therapy uses drugs to target specific genes or proteins to manage some types of breast cancer from developing and spreading. The human epidermal growth factor receptor 2 (HER2) is a gene involved in the development of breast cancer and Herceptin is a commonly used drug to target HER2-positive breast cancer [48]. Gene therapy utilizes virus to deliver and replicate new genes into patients' cells to replace damaged genes. This approach is a very selective targeted approach for precise molecular abnormalities associated with development of breast cancer, like mutated BRCA1 and p53 genes [49, 50].

Cancer stem cells (CSCs) are potential effectors of self-renewal, proliferation, and differentiation and play crucial roles in cancer survival and recurrence [51]. The necessity for cancer stem-cell therapy for breast cancer is justified by the recognition of stem cells in normal as well as in malignant tissues of the breast. CSCs have been identified as the source of molecular complexity of breast carcinoma in human. Thus, anti-CSC therapeutic approach would assist with prevention and management of various forms of cancer cells, including therapeutically resistant breast cancer cells by efficient targeting of breast CSC surface markers such as ESAþ, CD44þ, CD24−/low, Lineage- and ALDH1high [52, 53]. Owing to unpredictable physico-chemical properties of certain therapeutic agents in physiological environments, the exploitation of such targeted approaches, like the anti-CSC therapy, rests on the usage of suitable delivery systems. Nanomedicine offers the option of using specially designed drug-nanocarriers to integrally deliver therapeutic agents into cancer sites and CSCs niches [52]. Additionally, this option offers additional advantages including the designing of therapeutic systems directed towards pump-mediated drug resistant (ATP-driven) while having limited side effects on healthy cells and normal stem cells [52].

6. Photodynamic therapy for breast cancer

Photodynamic therapy (PDT) is a minimally invasive and clinically approved procedure for eradicating designated malignant cells with precise light activation of a non-toxic photochemotherapeutic agent, known as photosensitizer (PS). PDT is a

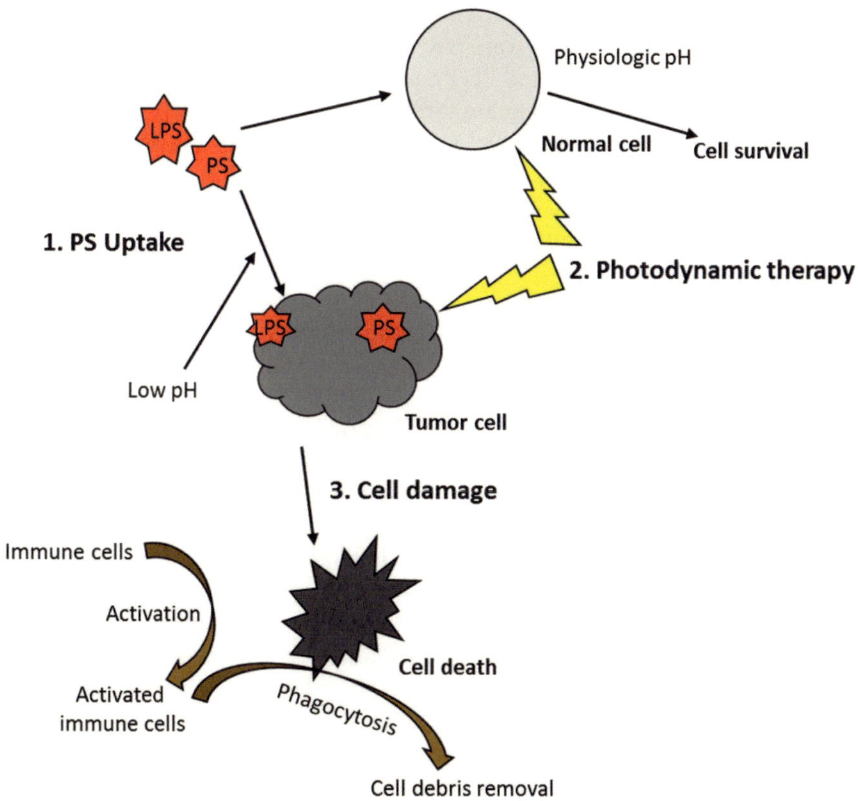

Figure 3.
Photodynamic cancer therapy actions: (1) administration and uptake of a photosensitizer (PS) and ligand-conjugated PS (LPS), which accumulate into either tumor cells/surrounding. The lower extracellular pH improves PS uptake by tumor cells. Conjugation of PS with specific ligands helps to target the vasculature surrounding breast tumor cells. (2) light irradiation at a wavelength matching the absorption properties of PS and (3) light activation of PS/LPS and induction of cell death. Immuno-activation stimulates phagocytosis of PDT-damaged tumor cells and cell removal. PDT may mediate an immune response causing tumor cell death at distant sites.

sequential procedure involving three main steps: (1) administration of a PS, which is internalized into either tumor cells or immediate vasculature; (2) local irradiation at a wavelength matching the absorbance peak of the PS; and (3) light activation of the PS, which mediates energy transfer cascades, generation of cytotoxic reactive oxygen species, and subsequent cell death [54, 55]. PDT is a selective approach and capable of using the specific traits of the tumor microenvironment of breast cancer. The low pH in tumor microenvironment enhances PS uptake into cells and this uptake can be further improved by conjugating PS to endothelial cell (EC)-specific ligands and target vasculature surrounding tumor (**Figure 3**). The effect of PDT is derived from three mechanisms: direct cytotoxic effects on tumor cells, indirect damage to tumor vasculature, and induction of immune responses [56]. Both parenchymal (tumor) and stromal (non-tumor) populations coexist in the tumor microenvironment, making it different from those of normal cells. There is a strong interrelation between these two populations within the tumor microenvironment as the ECs (which are stromal) are essential in providing the required hormones, oxygen, and other essential nutrients to both populations, while tumor cells develop and maintain the endothelial angiogenesis [57, 58]. PDT dosimetry depends on the complexity of the parenchymal cells and should take into consideration the stromal cells, so as to only attain complete tumor eradication [57]. Hence, the effective use of ligands for targeted PDT for breast cancer by conjugating factor VII (fVII) (ligand) with verteporfin or chlorin e6 (PSs) to exclusively prompt cell death mechanisms in the breast cancer cell population [59, 60]. Such approaches were efficient to target neovasculature and drug-resistant breast tumors, but paved the way for the improvement of future targeted PDT complexes [59–61]. The high recurrence and poor prognosis of breast cancer are directly related to the overexpression of certain receptors in breast cancer cells, such as estradiol receptors, the human epidermal growth factor receptor 2, gonadotropin-releasing hormone receptors, and tisular factor VII receptors [62]. They are appropriate sites for receptor-targeting approaches and beneficial for development of better PDT agents.

7. New photosensitizer-mediated PDT for breast cancer

The uptake and retention of PS by neoplastic cells is a decisive event in the progression and success of PDT. In its ground state, the singlet PS possesses two electrons with opposed spins. When irradiated at appropriate quantum energy (wavelength), the PS absorbs a photon and one of its electrons is excited into a higher energy level, which lasts for a few nanoseconds. The excited and unstable PS may lose the excess energy by fluorescing (light emission), internal conversion (heat emission), or undergoing intersystem crossing to reach a stable and excited triplet state with parallel spins and longer lifespan (microseconds). Due to the quantum selection rules, the triplet excited PS can interact and transfer its energy to molecular oxygen to form singlet oxygen (type II reaction, more common) or undergo electron transfer reactions to form reactive oxygen species (type I reaction) before returning to its ground state. The most common PSs are porphyrins, chlorins, bacteriochlorins, and phthalocyanines, they all possess tetrapyrrolic structures and many are clinically used. Phenothiazine, squaraine, and boron-dipyrromethene are major synthetic dyes, while hypericin, riboflavin, and curcumin are natural PSs. More and more PSs are being conjugated to antibodies, peptides, proteins, and other ligands for targeted PDT. Nanoparticles are multifunctional materials with various medical applications and they are mostly used in PDT to deliver PSs to the tumor-targeted sites, and recently to increase light penetration into tissue [63]. The increased use of nanoparticles as drug carriers significantly reduces the risk of non-specific accumulation and adverse effects in normal cells, while increases neoplastic targeting and therapeutic efficiency. Micelles, dendrimers, liposomes, and nanotubes are among the commonly used carrier systems in PDT. They do so by utilizing the enhanced permeability and retention effect and the acidic conditions created around the tumor microenvironment due to the high metabolic activities, developing porous endothelial junction and neovascularization [64, 65].

For the last two decades, extensive effort has been directed to the development of new PSs from first to third, and from simple to more complex PS entities for enhancing PDT outcomes in neoplastic-bearing animals and patients. Currently, third-generation PSs are under development in order to improve the PDT outcomes with two main research focuses, namely gene engineering-induced PDT and nano-medicine in PDT [66]. These PSs are synthesized based on specific cancerous characteristics like the Warburg effects, a recognized phenomenon arising due to the fact that cancer cells consume higher levels of glucose than normal cells. So, sugar-conjugated chlorin (glucose-chlorin) PSs which were synthesized showed improved cancer cell selective accumulation, induced immunogenic cell damage, and stronger antitumor effects than second-generation PSs. Such sugar-conjugated PSs induce very robust antitumor effects by targeting sugar receptors on the surface of cancer cells and tumor-associated macrophages in stromal cancer cells [67]. Other third-generation nanomaterial-mediated PSs like Chlorin E6 have shown strong ROS generation through formation of ion complexes. They are able to be encapsulated in gold nanoparticles as vesicles to achieve better penetration and are used for both diagnosis and treatment of cancer due to their strong absorption properties in the near-infrared range of 650–800 nm [68]. The cancer cell specificity and selectivity of PDT were inadequate with first- and second-generation PSs. With the development of third-generation PSs, PDT has become significantly beneficial for enhancing tumor targeting, tissue penetration depth, and therapeutic efficacy.

8. Conclusions

Breasts are well-developed organs in females for the production of milk during lactation. A special group of CDKs are required for proper breast cell cycle and functioning at all times. When the cell cycle is no longer under control, breast cancer begins to develop and is characterized by several breast morphological alternations, as well as chemical and pathophysiological changes. Various means of breast treatments are available and the targeted options seem to provide better therapeutic value than conventional therapies. PDT has emerged as an effective and potent breast cancer treatment; however, it is highly dependent on the development of more effective PSs. Thus, the development of new PSs is encouraged and PS complexes containing nanoparticles are one of the most recent developments to enhance delivery into tumor sites and treatment efficiency and decrease the adverse effects, which characterize the nontargeted therapies.

Acknowledgements

The work was conducted at the Laser Research Centre, Faculty of Health Sciences, University of Johannesburg, South Africa. The study was supported by the University Research Council of the University of Johannesburg. This work is based on the research supported by the South African Research Chairs Initiative of the Department of Science and Technology and National Research Foundation of South Africa (Grant No 98337), and the African Laser Centre.

Conflict of interest

The authors report no conflict of interest in this work.

Future directives

In relation to PDT being utilized as an alternative treatment therapy for breast cancer, further research is required for the development of targeted third-generation PSs as drug carriers in order to enhance the effectiveness of this treatment, as well as for investigating the upregulation of BRCA1 and BRCA2 breast cancer tumor suppressor genes in order to prevent changes in genetic materials and so their eradication.

Author details

Ivan Sosthene Mfouo Tynga* and Heidi Abrahamse
Laser Research Centre, Faculty of Health Sciences, University of Johannesburg, Doornfontein, South Africa

*Address all correspondence to: ivant@uj.ac.za

References

[1] Tanis P, Nieweg O, Olmos R, Kroon B. Anatomy and physiology of lymphatic drainage of the breast from the perspective of sentinel node biopsy. Journal of the American College of Surgeons. 2001;**192**:399-409

[2] Thomsen S, Tatman D. Physiological and pathological factors of human breast disease that can influence optical diagnosis. Annals of the New York Academy of Sciences. 1998;**838**(1):171-193

[3] Wood K, Cameron M, Fitzgerald K. Breast size, bra fit and thoracic pain in young women: A correlational study. Chiropractic & Osteopathy. 2008;**16**:1

[4] Wang JD, Levin PA. Metabolism, cell growth and the bacterial cell cycle. Nature Reviews. Microbiology. 2009;**7**(11):822-827

[5] Maton A, Lahart D, Hopkins J, Warner MQ, Johnson S, Wright JD. Cells: Building Blocks of Life. New Jersey: Prentice Hall; 1997. pp. 70-74. ISBN: 978-0-13-423476-2

[6] Wesierska-Gadek J, Gueorguieva M, Wojciechowski J, Horky M. Cell cycle arrest induced in human breast cancer cells by cyclin-dependent kinase inhibitors: A comparison of the effects exerted by roscovitine and olomoucine. Polish Journal of Pharmacology. 2004;**56**(5):635-641

[7] Loyer P, Trembley JH, Katona R, Kidd VJ, Lahti JM. Role of CDK/cyclin complexes in transcription and RNA splicing. Cellular Signalling. 2005;**17**(9):1033-1051

[8] Robbins SL, Cotran RS. In: Kumar V, Abbas AK, Fausto N, editors. Pathological Basis of Disease. Philadephia: PA. Elsevier; 2004. ISBN: 978-81-8147-528-2

[9] Lim S, Kaldis P. Cdks, cyclins and CKIs: Roles beyond cell cycle regulation. Development. 2013;**140**:3079-3093

[10] Landberg G, Roos G. The cell cycle in breast cancer. APMIS. 1997;**105**(8):575-589

[11] Nordqvist C. What you Need to Know about Breast Cancer. Medical New Today. 2017. Available from: https://www.medicalnewstoday.com/articles/37136.php [Retrieved: 12 October 2018]

[12] Champeris Tsaniras S, Kanellakis N, Symeonidou IE, Nikolopoulou P, Lygerou Z, Taraviras S. Licensing of DNA replication, cancer, pluripotency and differentiation: An interlinked world? Seminars in Cell & Developmental Biology. 2014;**30**:174-180

[13] National Breast Cancer Foundation. BRCA: The Breast Cancer Gene. Available from: https://www.nationalbreastcancer.org/what-is-brca [Retrieved: 03 November 2018]

[14] Sharma GN, Dave R, Sanadya J, Sharma P, Sharma KK. Various types and management of breast cancer: An overview. Journal of Advanced Pharmaceutical Technology & Research. 2010;**1**(2):109-126

[15] Akram M, Iqbal M, Daniyal M, Khan AU. Awareness and current knowledge of breast cancer. Biological Research. 2017;**50**:33

[16] Swietach P, Vaughan-Jones RD, Harris AL, Hulikova A. The chemistry, physiology and pathology of pH in cancer. Philosophical Transactions of the Royal Society of London. Series B, Biological Sciences. 2014;**369**(1638):20130099

[17] Wang S, Yan R, Zhang X, Chu Q, Shi Y. Molecular mechanism of pH-dependent substrate transport by an arginine-agmatine antiporter. PNAS. 2014;**111**(35):12734-12739

[18] Wike-Hooley JL, Haveman J, Reinhold HS. The relevance of tumour pH to the treatment of malignant disease. Radiotherapy and Oncology. 1984;**2**:343-366

[19] Gillies RJ, Liu Z, Bhujwalla Z. 31P-MRS measurements of extracellular pH of tumors using 3-aminopropylphosphonate. The American Journal of Physiology. 1994;**267**:C195-C203

[20] Tannock IF, Rotin D. Acid pH in tumors and its potential for therapeutic exploitation. Cancer Research. 1989;**49**:4373-4384

[21] Gusterson B, Warburton MJ, Mitchell D, Ellison M, Neville AM, Rudland PS. Distribution of myoepithelial cells and basement membrane proteins in the normal breast and in benign and malignant breast diseases. Cancer Research. 1982;**42**:4763-4770

[22] Hartwell L, Kastan M. Cell cycle control and cancer. Science. 1994;**266**:1821-1823

[23] Cavalieri E, Chakravarti D, Guttenplan J, Hart E, Ingle J, Jankowiak R, et al. Catechol estrogen quinones as initiators of breast and other human cancers: Implications for biomarkers of susceptibility and cancer prevention. Biochimica et Biophysica Acta. 2006;**1766**:63-68

[24] Jarde T, Perrier S, Vasson M, Caldefie-Chezet F. Molecular mechanisms of leptin and adiponectin in breast cancer. European Journal of Cancer. 2011;**47**:33-43

[25] Hanahan D, Weinberg R. The hallmarks of cancer. Cell. 2000;**100**:57-70

[26] Gupta G, Massagué J. Cancer metastasis: Building a framework. Cell. 2006;**127**:679-695

[27] Heim E, Valach L, Schaffner L. Coping and psychosocial adaptation: Longitudinal effects over time and stages in breast cancer. Psychosomatic Medicine. 1997;**59**:408-418

[28] Bednarek A, Sahin A, Brenner A, Johnston D, Aldaz C. Analysis of telomerase activity levels in breast cancer: Positive detection at the in situ breast carcinoma stage. Clinical Cancer Research. 1997;**3**(1):11-16

[29] Segal R, Evans W, Johnson D, Smith J, Colletta S, Gayton J. Structured exercise improves physical functioning in women with stages I and II breast cancer: Results of a randomized controlled trial. Journal of Clinical Oncology. 2001;**19**:657-665

[30] Moran M, Schnitt S, Giuliano A, Harris J, Khan S, Horton J. Society of surgical oncology–American society for radiation oncology consensus guideline on margins for breast-conserving surgery with whole-breast irradiation in stages I and II invasive breast cancer. International Journal of Radiation Oncology, Biology, Physics. 2014;**88**:553-564

[31] Jacquillat C, Weil M, Baillet F, Borel C, Auclerc G, Maublanc M. Results of neoadjuvant chemotherapy and radiation therapy in the breast-conserving treatment of 250 patients with all stages of infiltrative breast cancer. Cancer. 1990;**66**:119-129

[32] Neuman H, Morrogh M, Gonen M. Stage IV breast cancer in the era of targeted therapy, does surgery of the primary tumor matter. Cancer. 2015;**116**:1226-1233

[33] Lodha R, Nandeshwar S, Pal D. Risk factors for breast cancer among women in Bhopal urban agglomerate: A case-control study. Asian Pacific Journal of Cancer Prevention. 2011;**12**:2111-2115

[34] Houssami N, Turner R, Morrow M. Meta-analysis of pre-operative magnetic

resonance imaging (MRI) and surgical treatment for breast cancer. Breast Cancer Research and Treatment. 2017;**6**:1-11

[35] Fisher B, Anderson S, Redmond C, Cronin W. Reanalysis and results after 12 years of follow-up in a randomized clinical trial comparing total mastectomy with lumpectomy with or without irradiation in the treatment of breast cancer. The New England Journal of Medicine. 1995;**333**:1456-1461

[36] Yarnold J, Ashton A, Bliss J, Homewood J, Harper C, Hanson J. Fractionation sensitivity and dose response of late adverse effects in the breast after radiotherapy for early breast cancer: Long-term results of a randomised trial. Radiotherapy and Oncology. 2005;**75**:9-17

[37] Keskin G, Gumus A. Turkish hysterectomy and mastectomy patients-depression, body image, sexual problems and spouse relationships. Asian Pacific Journal of Cancer Prevention. 2011;**12**:425-432

[38] Keisch M, Vicini F, Kuske R, Hebert M, White J, Quiet C, et al. Initial clinical experience with the MammoSite breast brachytherapy applicator in women with early-stage breast cancer treated with breast-conserving therapy. International Journal of Radiation Oncology, Biology, Physics. 2003;**55**:289-293

[39] Osborne C, Yochmowitz M, Knight W, McGuire W. The value of estrogen and progesterone receptors in the treatment of breast cancer. Cancer. 1980;**46**:2884-2888

[40] Visvanathan K, Chlebowski R, Hurley P, Col F, Ropka M, Collyar D. American society of clinical oncology clinical practice guideline update on the use of pharmacologic interventions including tamoxifen, raloxifene, and aromatase inhibition for breast cancer risk reduction. Journal of Clinical Oncology. 2009;**27**:3235-3258

[41] Mehta S, Dhandapani K, De Sevilla L, Webb R, Mahesh V. Tamoxifen, a selective estrogen receptor modulator, reduces ischemic damage caused by middle cerebral artery occlusion in the ovariectomized female rat. Neuroendocrinology. 2003;**77**:44-50

[42] Riggs B, Hartmann L. Selective estrogen-receptor modulators—Mechanisms of action and application to clinical practice. The New England Journal of Medicine. 2003;**48**:618-629

[43] Vogel V, Costantino J, Wickerham D. Effects of tamoxifen vs raloxifene on the risk of developing invasive breast cancer and other disease outcomes: The NSABP study of tamoxifen and raloxifene (STAR) P-2 trial. JAMA. 2006;**295**:2727-2741

[44] Land S, Wickerham D, Costantino J. Patient-reported symptoms and quality of life during treatment with tamoxifen or raloxifene for breast cancer prevention: The NSABP study of Tamoxifen and Raloxifene (STAR) P-2 trial. JAMA. 2006;**295**:2742-2751

[45] Masood S. Neoadjuvant chemotherapy in breast cancers. Women's Health (London, England). 2016;**12**:480-491

[46] Benson I, Schrag D, Somerfield M, Cohen A, Figueredo A, Flynn P. American society of clinical oncology recommendations on adjuvant chemotherapy for stage II colon cancer. Journal of Clinical Oncology. 2004;**22**(16):3408-3419

[47] Shapiro C, Recht A. Side effects of adjuvant treatment of breast cancer. The New England Journal of Medicine. 2001;**344**:1997-2008

[48] Smith I, Procter M, Gelber RD, Guillaume S, Feyereislova A,

Dowsett M, et al. 2-year follow-up of trastuzumab after adjuvant chemotherapy in HER2-positive breast cancer: A randomised controlled trial. Lancet. 2007;**369**:29-36

[49] Liang Q, Li W, Zhao Z, Fu Q. Advancement of Wnt signal pathway and the target of breast cancer. Open Life Sciences. 2016;**11**:98-104

[50] Churpek JE, Marquez R, Neistadt B, Claussen K, Lee MK, Churpek MM, et al. Inherited mutations in cancer susceptibility genes are common among survivors of breast cancer who develop therapy-related leukemia. Cancer. 2016;**122**(2):304-311

[51] Teng YD, Wang L, Kabatas S, Ulrich H, Zafonte RD. Cancer stem cells or tumor survival cells? Stem Cells and Development. 2018;**27**(21):1466-1478

[52] Singh VK, Saini A, Chandra R. The implications and future perspectives of nanomedicine for cancer stem cell targeted therapies. Frontiers in Molecular Biosciences. 2017;**4**:52. DOI: 10.3389/fmolb.2017.00052

[53] Kakarala M, Wicha M. Implications of the cancer stem-cell hypothesis for breast cancer prevention and therapy. Journal of Clinical Oncology. 2008;**26**:2813-2820

[54] Płonka J, Latocha M. Photodynamic therapy in the treatment of breast cancer. Polski Merkuriusz Lekarski. 2012;**33**(195):173-175

[55] Master A, Livingston M, Sen Gupta A. Photodynamic nanomedicine in the treatment of solid tumors: Perspectives and challenges. Journal of Controlled Release. 2013;**168**(1):88-102

[56] Lamberti MJ, Vittar NBR, Rivarola VA. Breast cancer as photodynamic therapy target: Enhanced therapeutic efficiency by overview of tumor complexity. World Journal of Clinical Oncology. 2014;**5**(5):901-907

[57] Rumie Vittar NB, Lamberti MJ, Pansa MF, Vera RE, Rodriguez ME, Cogno IS, et al. Ecological photodynamic therapy: New trend to disrupt the intricate networks within tumor ecosystem. Biochimica et Biophysica Acta. 2013;**1835**:86-99

[58] Herbert SP, Stainier DY. Molecular control of endothelial cell behaviour during blood vessel morphogenesis. Nature Reviews. Molecular Cell Biology. 2011;**12**:551-564

[59] Hu Z, Rao B, Chen S, Duanmu J. Targeting tissue factor on tumour cells and angiogenic vascular endothelial cells by factor VII-targeted verteporfin photodynamic therapy for breast cancer in vitro and in vivo in mice. BMC Cancer. 2010;**10**:235

[60] Duanmu J, Cheng J, Xu J, Booth CJ, Hu Z. Effective treatment of chemoresistant breast cancer in vitro and in vivo by a factor VII-targeted photodynamic therapy. British Journal of Cancer. 2011;**104**:1401-1409

[61] Thomas N, Pernot M, Vanderesse R, Becuwe P, Kamarulzaman E, Da Silva D, et al. Photodynamic therapy targeting neuropilin-1: Interest of pseudopeptides with improved stability properties. Biochemical Pharmacology. 2010;**80**:226-235

[62] Oude Munnink TH, Nagengast WB, Brouwers AH, Schröder CP, Hospers GA, Lub-de Hooge MN, et al. Molecular imaging of breast cancer. Breast. 2009;**18**(Suppl 3):S66-S73

[63] Abrahamse H, Hamblin MR. New photosensitizers for photodynamic therapy. The Biochemical Journal. 2016;**473**(4):347-364

[64] Khodabandehloo H, Zahednasab H, Hafez AA. Nanocarriers usage for drug delivery in Cancer therapy. Iranian Journal of Cancer Prevention. 2016;**9**:e3966-e3973

[65] Egusquiaguirre SP, Igartua M, Hernández RM, Pedraz JL. Nanoparticle delivery systems for cancer therapy: Advances in clinical and preclinical research. Clinical & Translational Oncology. 2012;**14**:83-93

[66] Kou J, Dou D, Yang L. Porphyrin photosensitizers in photodynamic therapy and its applications. Oncotarget. 2017;**8**(46):81591-81603

[67] Kataoka H, Nishie H, Hayashi N, Tanaka M, Nomoto A, Yano S, et al. New photodynamic therapy with next-generation photosensitizers. Annals of Translational Medicine. 2017;**5**(8):183-190

[68] Lin J, Wang S, Huang P, Wang Z, Chen S, Niu G, et al. Photosensitizer-loaded gold vesicles with strong plasmonic coupling effect for imaging-guided photothermal/photodynamic therapy. ACS Nano. 2013;7:5320-5329

Section 4

Diet, Exercise and Other Lifestyle Factors for Breast Cancer Prevention

Chapter 6

Breast Cancer and Exercise

Deniz Kocamaz and Tülin Düger

Abstract

Breast cancer is the most common type of cancer and the leading cause of death in women. Chemotherapy drugs, which are used to suppress growth and proliferation of cancer cells, prevent or minimize treatment-related symptoms, and improve the quality of life, lead to the destruction of normal cells with therapeutic effects as well as toxic effects. In response, symptoms such as pain, nausea, vomiting, fatigue, anorexia, anxiety, and depression occur in patients. Chemotherapy and its side effects adversely affect the physical and functional capacity of patients with cancer. In particular, the decrease in aerobic capacity affects muscle strength, endurance body awareness, and the quality of life. The practice of aerobic exercise programs during the treatment of breast cancer is important for reducing the side effects, improving physiological health, improving physical functions, preventing weight gain, and maintaining muscle strength. When the rehabilitation programs for breast cancer are individualized, become specific, and realistic goals are set, the positive effects of exercise can be seen.

Keywords: breast cancer, exercise, aerobic exercise, physiotherapy, rehabilitation

1. Introduction

Breast cancer is the most common type of cancer in women. The incidence of breast cancer is increasing all over the world. The mortality rate of breast cancer decreases in developed countries in parallel with the methods used for diagnosis and treatment, but the rate of breast cancer mortality increases in developing countries [1].

Different treatment methods can be used in breast cancer treatment. Treatment protocols, which are suitable for surgical, radiotherapy, and systematic, can be practiced individually or after one another. While the treatment programs are being developed, the importance of improving the survivability and the quality of life as well as the control of cancer-related symptoms are increasing [2, 3].

Chemotherapy drugs are used in cancer cells to suppress growth and proliferation, to prevent or minimize treatment-related symptoms, and to improve quality of life. However, these drugs, along with their therapeutic and toxic effects, destroy normal cells. Fatigue, loss of appetite, nausea, vomiting, pain, weakness, hair loss, bone marrow suppression, insomnia, mucosal and skin problems, pain, neurological problems, and sexual problems may occur depending on the medication taken after chemotherapy and the tolerance of the individual [4].

During chemotherapy and rehabilitation process of patients, systemic problems, laboratory values, and high fever should be evaluated before and after each treatment session. The patient can continue the exercise program, if the fever is below 38°C, the platelet count is 50, 000 and above, the leukocyte count is 5000-10,000, and the hemoglobin is 8 or above. Besides, symptoms such as nausea, vomiting, and diarrhea should be taken into consideration regarding the quality of the exercise program. The minimal changes in these values lead to differences in the type, severity, and duration of the exercise program [3].

Radiotherapy is one of the preferred methods for the treatment of breast cancer. In the radiotherapy process, skin damage, sensory problems, loss of joint mobility, and bone fracture risk should be taken into consideration, while planning rehabilitation programs. In addition, changes in normal tissue exposed to radiation cause some side effects. Some of these side effects are as follows: fatigue, bone marrow depression, erythema in the skin, pigmentation, burns, hair loss, central nervous system effects, bone growth retardation, radiation pneumonia, pain, and ulcers. When planning rehabilitation programs in patients receiving radiotherapy, it should be aimed to minimize the possible side effects of the treatment and to increase the functionality level of individuals [5].

Patients admitted to oncology outpatient clinics, hormone therapy, chemotherapy, and radiotherapy can experience problems depending on the side effects of drugs. Increasing the quality of life of individuals and minimizing the side effects of treatment is one of the priorities of the health care members working in the field of oncology.

2. Breast cancer and quality of life

Cancer is a chronic disease that has physical, psychological, and cognitive recovery and aggravation periods. About 33% of cancer survivors reported that the obvious cause of deterioration in the quality of life is fatigue. The primary goal of women with breast cancer and survivors of breast cancer is the improvement of functions affected by cancer-related treatments [6].

The period after diagnosis and treatment means the important adaptations concerning physical, social, cognitive, emotional, and economic aspects for the patients with breast cancer and their immediate circle. The activity participation levels, interests, and quality of life of individuals are reshaped, especially for the survivors. The goals of rehabilitation vary in cancer patients at different stages of the disease. The primary goal is to continue and maintain the quality of life and functionality in the diagnosis phase. It is in the forefront to support improvement in the treatment stage and to prevent the quality of life to be adversely affected. The inclusion of individual submaximal aerobic exercise programs to maintain and enhance the quality of life is the first step in oncologic rehabilitation.

Various scales have been developed to determine the quality of life in breast cancer. Nowadays, there is growing evidence that quality of life in breast cancer should be evaluated in detail. Besides being affected by many factors, the quality of life is subjective and difficult to evaluate. There are few specific questionnaire for cancer: European Organization for Research and Treatment of Cancer (EORTC) Quality of Life Questionnaire and Breast Cancer Supplement (EORTC QLQ—C 30 and QLQ—BR 23), The Functional Assessment of Chronic İllness Therapy General Questionnaire and its Breast Cancer Supplement (FACIT-G and FACIT-B), and The Breast Cancer Chemotherapy Questionnaire (BCQ) [7, 8].

3. Breast cancer and functional capacity

The long process and the side effects of cancer treatment may lead to a decrease in functional capacity. It might lead particularly to the reduction of aerobic capacity, muscle strength reduction, flexibility, changes in body composition, and affecting patients' health-related quality of life. In recent years, breast cancer mortality is decreasing. However, the need for rehabilitation in the recovery of the reduction in functional capacity due to the side effects of the treatment is increasing [9].

Aerobic exercises, stretching, relaxation exercises, strengthening exercises, combined exercise programs, body awareness training, energy conservation techniques, dance therapy, and yoga are aimed to increase functional capacity in breast cancer patients [10].

Individualized rehabilitation programs should be planned to determine exercise capacity and increase functional capacity in cancer patients. A 6-minute walk test, bicycle ergometer, and walking band can be used under the supervision of physiotherapist with cardiologist recommendation during the evaluation and exercise training.

4. Breast cancer and rehabilitation

Cancer rehabilitation in the literature is one of the special rehabilitation approaches in physiotherapy and rehabilitation since 1940. In a study conducted in 1978, the areas where rehabilitation was needed were investigated, and problems were identified in the areas of psychological stress, pain, muscle weakness, daily life activities, ambulation, and family support. Thus, the studies aimed to support the quality of life of cancer patients have gained importance [3].

Currently, studies conducted with cancer patients indicated the impact of exercise on fatigue, pain, muscle strength, functional capacity, and quality of life. Due to cancer treatments and its side effects, changes in physical, functional, cognitive, and emotional well-being may be observed in patients. This situation affects the daily activities and role functions of the cancer patients and clearly emphasizes the need for rehabilitation programs [10].

Fatigue is the most common symptom in cancer patients. The National Comprehensive Cancer Network has expressed the relationship between fatigue and cancer as a result of the psychosocial interaction of physical, systematic, cognitive, and emotional changes due to long-term treatment. The main purpose of oncologic rehabilitation is to remove the chemicals taken by systemic treatments and radiotherapy, increase the amount of tissues oxygenation, and maintain muscle strength and endurance. Aerobic exercises have an important role in accelerating the excretion of toxic substances accumulated in the body due to the side effects of radiotherapy and chemotherapy and increasing the oxygenation of tissues in order to minimize fatigue complaints [11, 12].

4.1 Breast cancer and oncologic rehabilitation

Oncologic rehabilitation is a medical process that aims to reduce the cancer patients' complaints during the illness, to increase the level of independence, and to increase the quality of life. Studies on conservation, recovery, and development of the physical, environmental, social, cognitive, psychological, and professional functions require experience and multidisciplinary team in the field of oncological rehabilitation. The oncologic rehabilitation team consists of patients, doctors, nurses, physiotherapists, psychologists, nutritionists, dieticians, social workers, speech therapists, and relatives of the patient. Physiotherapists aim to improve the quality of life of cancer patients using individualized exercise programs in the treatment and survival periods starting from the diagnosis stage [12, 13].

While planning individual exercise training in oncologic rehabilitation, the type and stage of cancer, as well as the patient's complaints, should be considered. Progressive weighing down should be performed to increase muscle performance. This weigh principle means increasing the frequency, intensity, severity, and exercise type gradually and individually. It aims to maximize the cardiopulmonary potential with pretreatment term exercises in cancer. In the treatment term, the aim is to improve the quality of life, the functional capacity of the individual, and to develop their limited skills. In the posttreatment term, the aim of exercise training is to adapt the individual to the physical and environmental changes that may occur in daily life.

The survival duration of breast cancer patients increased due to the developments in cancer treatments. It is important to decrease the treatment-related complications and improve the quality of life during the survival period. Upper extremity limitations, pain, fatigue, sensory problems, the decrease in functional capacity, and loss of muscle strength are common complications in breast cancer patients. In the studies conducted in the field of oncologic rehabilitation with breast cancer patients, it was stated that aerobic exercise programs had an important role in increasing the quality of life and functionality. Furthermore, in the literature, the effects of various physiotherapy applications such as pilates and yoga exercises, complex decongestive physiotherapy applications, strengthening exercises, relaxation exercises, and banding techniques have been shown within the scope of oncologic rehabilitation programs for individuals with breast cancer [14].

4.2 Stretching and relaxation exercises in breast cancer

Stretching exercises are frequently preferred in physiotherapy and rehabilitation programs, and they are a simple but effective component of treatment when applied correctly. Although the literature on stretching exercises is constantly being updated, physiotherapists are used to improve normal joint movement and physical fitness to reduce muscular fatigue and to improve proprioception and body perception.

Exercises consisting of active stretching and relaxation techniques such as pilates, yoga, and dance therapy can be used in rehabilitation programs in breast cancer patients. These exercises are preferred to support the body image of the individual during the treatment and posttreatment periods, to increase awareness, and to improve the physical fitness of the patient. It is aimed to accelerate the excretion of toxic substances and reduce fatigue complaints by increasing the circulation and muscle feeding with stretching and relaxation exercises [10, 15].

4.3 Aerobic exercise in breast cancer

Aerobic capacity refers to the measurement of the functional capacity of the cardiopulmonary system. It is associated with the ability to perform dynamic, medium/high-intensity exercise, which includes the use of long-term, large muscle groups. Aerobic exercises contribute to increase the quality of life by decreasing the fatigue level due to cancer treatment and insulin resistance due to the metabolic structure of the individual with breast cancer [16].

Aerobic exercise training means increasing the energy capacity of the muscle with exercise. Exercise programs are usually prepared considering the frequency, duration, density, and type parameters. The intensity of aerobic exercise progresses from low to medium in breast cancer patients. The heart rate should be 65–80%, and the exercise program should continue for at least 20–30 minutes for the minimum effect [10, 16].

Increasing the level of physical activity in cancer contributes to increase survival rates and quality of life. It has been shown that the mortality rate decreases with regular exercise programs in individuals with breast cancer. Increasing physical activity during breast cancer treatment has an important role in minimizing the side effects of chemotherapy and radiotherapy, providing body awareness, and increasing muscle strength [17, 18].

Physiological responses following aerobic exercise training result in changes in the cardiovascular system and peripheral muscles. With regular aerobic exercise, the capacity to use oxygen in peripheral muscles increases. In addition to endurance exercises, change in oxidative enzyme capacity, fiber type, and capillary density is observed. Lactate accumulation in muscle is reduced, and less carbon dioxide production is achieved during the exercise process. Maximal oxygen consumption, one of the side effects of cancer treatments, decreased, and accumulation of toxic substances causing fatigue complaints increased.

In studies on the effectiveness of aerobic exercise in breast cancer patients and survivors, it was stated that myoglobin levels increased, immune system functions improved, fat destruction was accelerated, functional capacity and quality of life improved, and body composition improved, besides the reduction of fatigue complaints and acceleration of the excretion of toxic substances. In addition, red blood cell counts may decrease in cancer patients as one of the side effects of treatment. This leads to a reduction in physical performance and fatigue, as oxygen requirements cannot be fully met in activities requiring low effort. For this reason, the exercise programs must be personal. The severity of the exercise must adjusted according to personeal needs and the physiological responses. These details are important for cancer rehabilitation [18, 19].

Aerobic exercises in breast cancer patients have been proven to support body image and self-esteem, increase physical performance, weight control, and muscle strength. It is known that the aerobic exercises performed during the chemotherapy period contribute to the reduction of complaints due to side effects and to increase the functional capacity and quality of life. Nowadays, in the field of oncologic rehabilitation, the need for studies involving exercise programs during different treatments in breast cancer patients is increasing.

4.4 Calisthenic exercise in breast cancer

The word kalistenik is of Greek origin and derived from the word sthenos, which means kallos, and force, which means beauty. It is defined as the art of using your body to improve human physics. Calisthenic exercise is a useful form of exercise because the major muscle groups can be used in paced, rhythmic, different time, number, and intensity, which can be modified and can meet different physical fitness parameters. It can be applied without equipment. These aerobic exercises, which can be used for durability and flexibility, have been shaped by the modification of the Carlson Fatigue Curve test [20].

Calisthenic exercises are preferred because of objective evaluation of physical performance, compliance with home exercise programs, and safe application to individuals with chronic disease. The advantage of these exercises is that they can be modified according to the individual and contributes to balance, strength, agility, coordination, and endurance.

Calisthenic exercise practice principles

- It is recommended that these exercises be performed in a noise-free environment and accompanied by music.

- It is suitable to be rhythmic and counted in order to contribute to the aerobic capacity.
- For the 30-minute program, 1–3 exercises should be selected for each category for prone, prone and side-lying, sitting, standing categories, and 60 minutes for each category.
- The exercise program should be performed at the same time throughout the treatment, preferably in the morning.
- Calisthenic exercises can be performed individually or in groups.

Calisthenic exercises in breast cancer patients can be preferred safely in diagnosis, treatment, and survival stages. Exercise examples that can be applied in breast cancer patients are as follows. These exercises should be applied gradually with the principle of individual weighing and under the supervision of a physiotherapist.

1. Reciprocal hip flexion and extension in the supine position.
2. Lifting reciprocal flat leg in the supine lying position.
3. Setting up a bridge in the supine position.
4. Hip abduction in the lateral lying position.
5. Beck extension in the prone position.
6. Shoulder elevation in sitting position.
7. The circular movement of the shoulders from the front to the back in sitting position.
8. Scapula adduction in sitting position (hands on back).
9. Shoulder flexion in standing position.
10. Shoulder abduction in standing position.
11. Reciprocal lateral flexion of the trunk in standing position.
12. Upward movement on toes with arm up.
13. Reciprocal hip and knee flexion in standing position.
14. Half-squat in standing position [16].

4.5 Strengthening exercises in breast cancer

Muscle strength is the force that a muscle or muscle group spends against resistance with maximum effort. Strengthening exercises preferred in women with breast cancer to protect and improve the muscular force of the vertebrae and extremities, to improve endurance, increase function and develop the quality of life. Progressive resistant exercise is a method that strengthens the muscle according to the principles of adaptation and weighing down. DeLorme and Oxford techniques are commonly used methods in progressive resistant exercise.

Reduction in bone density, fatigue, decreasing of physical activity as a result of the loss of energy, decrease in the participation of Type I muscle fibers in contraction and loss of strength, anxiety, and depression may be observed depending on the side effects of breast cancer treatments. Strengthening exercises are required to increase muscle function and exercise capacity. In the literature, the most commonly used strengthening exercises in breast cancer patients are progressive resistant exercises. Schmitz et al. reported that there was a 30–50% increase in muscle strength in breast cancer patients who participated in progressive resistance exercise programs for 2 days and 12 months [21, 22].

In oncologic rehabilitation, exercise is recommended for 12 weeks, 3 times a week, 65–80% of the maximum heart rate, and 4–6 severity on the Borg scale. It is important to not to increase the fatigue complaints and maintain the physical performance of breast cancer patients during the strengthening exercises. It is important to not to exercise more than 3 days a week and to plan 1-day exercise and 1-day rest (can be 2 day rest interval according to patient tolerance) for breast cancer patients.

5. Disease process and exercise

The World Health Organization mandates that exercise repairs physical, physiological, and mental wellbeing in general and that consistent moderate-intensity exercise decreases the risk of cardiovascular disease, diabetes, and cancer [23]. Exercise programs for breast cancer have been reported to contribute to positive outcomes with developed treatment methods [24].

When creating rehabilitation programs, the type and stage of cancer, the needs and expectations of the individual, the progression of the disease, the status of the metastasis, the treatment protocols, and the side effects of the treatment should be considered. Physiotherapists who have an important role in the team of rehabilitation should take a holistic approach to pre/post (remission) treatment periods, active care, protection, and palliative periods.

Determining the duration and frequency of rest intervals in planning the exercise programs that include individual loading principles increases the success of physiotherapy and rehabilitation in parallel with the process of the disease in reducing the fatigue complaints [25].

5.1 Pretreatment period in breast cancer

The pretreatment period is the process in which the disease is recognized by the breast cancer patient. The patient is admitted to the hospital, the diagnosis is made, but the treatments are not started yet. It is a sensitive and anxious period for the patients, and the physiotherapist's approach to the patient is important for the effectiveness of the treatment. All body systems should be evaluated. The functional status should be determined prior to the treatments, and the effects of the treatments should be demonstrated. Patients and their relatives should be informed about the importance of the starting physiotherapy programs during treatments, survival period, and in the palliative period [3, 26]. The exercises recommended during this period are given in **Figure 1**.

Studies in recent years have shown that exercise, especially moderate-intensity aerobic exercise, has been noted to be advantageous in some studies regarding the breast cancer outcomes, decreasing the mortality rate by >30%, and decreasing recurrence rates for females following a breast cancer diagnosis [27].

Exercise Type: Aerobic exercises
Exercise Propospal: Walking, Swimming, Cailsthenic and Strengthening Exercises
Exercise Intensity: 65-80% of the maximum heart rate
Moderate - 4-6 severity on the Borg scale
Exercise Frequency: 3-4 days a week

Figure 1.
Exercise recommendation in pretreatment period.

5.2 Treatment period in breast cancer (active term)

It is the period when the treatments started, continued in the breast cancer patient, and the side effects started to be observed. All systems in patients receiving chemotherapy and radiotherapy should be evaluated in detail at frequent intervals. Evaluating and recording the fatigue and pain are important in this period. Functional disability and endurance loss should be considered in planning treatment programs.

Focusing on physiotherapy and rehabilitation programs during the treatment period will enable the patients to adapt to the new period of cancer. Starting the exercise programs at the submaximal level will improve the quality of life of individuals and facilitate their adaptation to treatment by taking into account the side effects that may occur following the first dose of treatment. In the literature, it was stated that it would be effective to give aerobic exercises beginning from the active period in breast cancer patients receiving chemotherapy and radiotherapy [5, 28, 29]. The exercises recommended during this period are presented in **Figure 2**.

In the recent studies, it has been shown that respirator and functional capacity are increased, and sleeping disturbance, mood disturbance, and anxiety decreased following a 12-week aerobic exercise program in women undergoing adjuvant chemotherapy [30].

5.3 Maintenance/protection period in breast cancer

The exercise of maintenance and protection period consists of long-term exercises to keep the disease in remission. All systems and circumstances, caused by side effects, should be evaluated in detail at frequent intervals. Findings of different treatments should be noted. Complications such as muscle weakness and posture problems should be considered when planning physiotherapy and rehabilitation programs.

Ongoing physiotherapy rehabilitation studies are needed for women with breast cancer, especially during chemotherapy. Individualized exercise programs are the

Exercise Type: Aerobic Exercises, Body Awarness Exercise
Exercise Propospal: Walking, Swimming, Cailsthenic Exercises, Pilates, Yoga, Respiratory Exercises, Stretching And Relaxation Exercises, Posture Exercise
Exercise Intensity: 40-60% of the maximum heart rate
Mild exercises
Exercise Frequency: 3 days a week
Exercise Duration: 45-60 minutes (rest intervals should be long).

Figure 2.
Exercise recommendation in treatment period.

important parts of the breast cancer treatment in order to reduce the side effects of treatment, to support individuals from physical, functional, and cognitive aspects, and to improve the quality of life [25]. The exercises recommended for this period are presented in **Figure 3**.

5.4 Posttreatment period/remission period in breast cancer

Remission period refers to the survival period in which cancer treatments are completed. All systems should be evaluated in detail. Musculoskeletal problems, sensory, motor, and cognitive problems should be examined in detail. When creating physiotherapy and rehabilitation programs, the individual's specific needs and complaints should be taken into consideration. Loss of muscle strength, poor posture, loss of endurance, and decrease in quality of life are the most common complaints.

Most of the studies related to the breast cancer patients are concerned with the survival period. The effects of aerobic exercises especially on body image, sexual functions, quality of life, functional capacity, and cognitive functions have been confirmed [6, 10, 11]. The exercises recommended during this period are given in **Figure 4**.

In a cohort-longitudinal study, it was observed that fast walking (3 h/week) prior to and following a breast cancer diagnosis in postmenopausal women reduced the mortality rate by 40% [31]. Most importantly, reports in previous systematic reviews suggested that aerobic exercise with moderate-high intensity (50–85% of maximal heart rate), 3 times/week ranging between 8 and 24 weeks, to be the most frequent mode for breast cancer patients and survivors. Similarly, this program may also have a positive effect on the cardiovascular, muscular, and neurological systems. As a consequence, this can lead to improvements in quality of life, such as the ability to deal with daily tasks [32].

Exercise Type: Aerobic Exercises

Exercise Propospal: Walking, Swimming, Cailsthenic and Strengthening Exercises, Posture Exercise

Exercise Intensity: 65-75% of the maximum heart rate

Moderate - 4-6 severity on the Borg scale

Exercise Frequency: 3-4 days a week

Exercise Duration: 45-60 minute

Figure 3.
Exercise recommendation in maintenance/protection period.

Exercise Type: Aerobic Exercises

Exercise Propospal: Walking, Swimming, Cycling, Progressive Exercises, Posture Exercise

Exercise Intensity: 65-75% of the maximum heart rate

Moderate - 4-6 severity on the Borg scale

Exercise Frequency: 3-4 days a week

Exercise Duration: 45-60 minutes

Figure 4.
Exercise recommendation in posttreatment period.

Exercise Type: Aerobic Exercises, Daily Life Activities

Exercise Propospal: Normal joint motions, Daily life activities, respiratory exercise, Walking

Exercise Intensity: 40-60% of the maximum heart rate

Mild exercises

Exercise Frequency: 3 days a week

Exercise Duration: 45-60 minutes (rest intervals should be long).

Figure 5.
Exercise recommendation in palliative period.

5.5 Palliative period in breast cancer

According to the definition of the World Health Organization, palliative care is the time when someone is facing a life-threatening illness. It is an approach used to improve the quality of life of patients and their relatives. In this period, rehabilitation programs should be planned considering physical, psychosocial, and mental problems, especially pain. The disability and activity limitations of the body structure and function of individuals should be focused. Improvable/curable functions and the specific needs of the patient are important. Increased muscle strength and locomotor skills should be maintained. Physiotherapy and rehabilitation programs should include daily living activities and the use of ancillary equipment during this period. For this purpose, physiotherapists should determine the need for support equipment and be involved in the adaptation process of the individual and provide the necessary training [3, 33]. The exercise recommendation for this period is given in **Figure 5**.

6. Conclusion/summary

Breast cancer is the most common type of cancer among women in the world. The increase in the average lifetime, the change in lifestyle, the spread of screening studies, and the increase in the notification of cancer cases can be considered as the main reasons for the increase in the incidence of breast cancer. Long-term treatment and side effects in breast cancer cause decreasing in the functional capacity of the individual with cancer. Particularly, the decrease in aerobic capacity negatively affects muscle strength, endurance, and body perception, leading to a decrease in quality of life. Besides, symptoms such as systemic problems, blood values results, and high fever during chemotherapy may cause change in the type, duration, severity, and mobilization status of the exercise programs. The practice of aerobic exercise programs during the treatment of breast cancer is important in reducing the side effects, improving physiological health, improving physical functions, and preventing weight gain and maintaining muscle strength. Rehabilitation in breast cancer contributes to the restoration of the problems caused by the disease and its treatment, keeping physical, psychosocial, and occupational functions at the highest level. In women with breast cancer, rehabilitation programs including aerobic exercises are in parallel with the stage of the disease and the treatment process. Also, increasing physical activity level and functional capacity is an important approach in coping with the disease process.

As a result, although there are very important developments in cancer prevention and early diagnosis and treatment methods, a breast cancer diagnosis is rapidly increasing in the world. Cancer patients at the stage of diagnosis continue their daily life routine; they have a high functional level, and they have no side effects. For this reason, many cancer patients state that the quality of life decreases with the onset of treatments, fatigue, long-term hospitalizations, repeated scans, and the effect of drug treatment. Satisfactory and effective applications are needed to maintain the functional status and quality of life of breast cancer patients. Oncologic rehabilitation approaches should be planned and implemented as individual programs adapted to the patients following a comprehensive evaluation of breast cancer patients. Individual rehabilitation programs can be planned as aerobic exercises, pulmonary rehabilitation, body awareness training, and cognitive rehabilitation. It is aimed to maximize the quality of life, minimize complaints, and increase functional capacity with exercise programs in breast cancer patients. More specifically, studies on the appropriate exercise program for breast cancer are needed with a clearer and more comprehensive analysis of the functional capacity and quality of life that are anticipated for positive health outcomes.

Acknowledgements

We would like to thank our esteemed patients we met during the studies we have carried out in the field of oncologic rehabilitation.

Author details

Deniz Kocamaz[1]* and Tülin Düger[2]

1 Faculty of Health Science, Department of Physiotherapy and Rehabilitation, Hasan Kalyoncu University, Gaziantep, Turkey

2 Faculty of Health Science, Department of Physiotherapy and Rehabilitation, Hacettepe University, Ankara, Turkey

*Address all correspondence to: denizerdan@gmail.com

References

[1] Jemal A, Bray F, Center M, Ferlay J, Ward E, Forman D. Global cancer statistics. CA: A Cancer Journal for Clinicians. 2011;**61**(2):69-90

[2] Bancroft MI. Physiotherapy in cancer rehabilitation: a theoretical approach. Physiotherapy. 2003;**89**(12):729-733

[3] Düger T, Atasavun, Uysal S. Kanser Rehabilitasyonu. In: Karaduman AYTÖ, editor. Fizyoterapi Rehabilitasyon. Ankara: Pelikan Yayıncılık; 2016. pp. 505-517

[4] Whelan TJ, Pignol J-P, Levine MN, Julian JA, MacKenzie R, Parpia S, et al. Long-term results of hypofractionated radiation therapy for breast cancer. New England Journal of Medicine. 2010;**362**(6):513-520

[5] Cuzick J. Radiotherapy for breast cancer. Journal of the National Cancer Institute. 2005;**97**(6):406-407

[6] Bower J, Garet D, Sternlieb B, Ganz P, Irwin M, Olmstead R, et al. Yoga for persistent fatigue in breast cancer survivors. Cancer. 2012;**118**(15):3766-3775

[7] Lemieux J, Goodwin PJ, Bordeleau LJ, Lauzier S, Théberge V. Quality-of-life measurement in randomized clinical trials in breast cancer: an updated systematic review (2001-2009). Journal of the National Cancer Institute. 2011;**103**(3):178-231

[8] Montazeri A. Health-related quality of life in breast cancer patients: a bibliographic review of the literature from 1974 to 2007. Journal of Experimental & Clinical Cancer Research. 2008;**27**(1):32

[9] Travier N, Velthuis MJ, Bisschop CNS, van den Buijs B, Monninkhof EM, Backx F, et al. Effects of an 18-week exercise programme started early during breast cancer treatment: a randomised controlled trial. BMC Medicine. 2015;**13**(1):121

[10] Vardar Yağlı N, Şener G, Arıkan H, Sağlam M, İnal İnce D, Savcı S, et al. Do yoga and aerobic exercise training have impact on functional capacity, fatigue, peripheral muscle strength, and quality of life in breast cancer survivors? Integrative Cancer Therapies. 2015;**14**(2):125-132

[11] McNeely M, Campbell K, Rowe B, Klassen T, Mackey J, Courneya K. Effects of exercise on breast cancer patients and survivors: a systematic review and meta-analysis. Canadian Medical Association Journal. 2006;**175**(1):34-41

[12] Irwin ML. Physical activity interventions for cancer survivors. British Journal of Sports Medicine. 2009;**43**(1):32-38

[13] Keser İ, Özdemİr K, Ertürk B, Haspolat M, Duman T, Esmer M. Kanser hastalarina yönelik onkolojik fizyoterapi ve rehabilitasyon ünitesi'nde sunulan hizmetlerin analizi. Gazi Üniversitesi Sağlık Bilimleri Dergisi. 2017;**1**(1):18-27

[14] McNeely ML, Campbell K, Ospina M, Rowe BH, Dabbs K, Klassen TP, et al. Exercise interventions for upper-limb dysfunction due to breast cancer treatment. Cochrane Database of Systematic Reviews. 2010;(6)

[15] Spence RR, Heesch KC, Brown WJ. Exercise and cancer rehabilitation: a systematic review. Cancer Treatment Reviews. 2010;**36**(2):185-194

[16] Kocamaz D, Düger T. Meme Kanserli Kadınlarda Farklı Tedaviler ile Birlikte Verilen Kalistenik Egzersizlerin Fiziksel Aktivite Düzeyi ve Depresyona Etkisi. Türk Fizyoterapi ve Rehabilitasyon Dergisi. 2017;**28**(3):93-99

[17] Chen X, Zheng Y, Zheng W, Gu K, Chen Z, Lu W, et al. The effect of regular exercise on quality of life among breast cancer survivors. American Journal of Epidemiology. 2009;**170**(7):854-862

[18] Fobair P, Stewart SL, Chang S, D'onofrio C, Banks PJ, Bloom JR. Body image and sexual problems in young women with breast cancer. Psycho-Oncology. 2006;**15**(7):579-594

[19] Fong D, Ho J, Hui B, Lee A, Macfarlane D, Leung S. Physical activity for cancer survivors: meta-analysis of randomised controlled trials. BMJ. 2012;**344**:370

[20] Adams RC. Rehabilitation Calisthenics. Games, Sports and Exercises for Physically Handycapped; 1979. p. 411

[21] Courneya K, Segal R, Mackey J, Gelmon K, Reid R, Friedenreich C, et al. Effects of aerobic and resistance exercise in breast cancer patients receiving adjuvant chemotherapy: a multicenter randomized controlled trial. Journal of Clinical Oncology. 2007;**25**(28):4396-4404

[22] Cheema B, Gaul C, Lane K, Singh M. Progressive resistance training in breast cancer: a systematic review of clinical trials. Breast Cancer Research and Treatment. 2008;**109**(1):9-26

[23] http://apps.who.int/iris/bitstream/10665/43035/1/9241592222_eng.pdf?ua=1

[24] Singh B, Spence RR, Steele ML, Sandler CX, Peake JM, Hayes SC. A systematic review and meta-analysis of the safety, feasibility and effect of exercise in women with stage II+ breast cancer. Archives of Physical Medicine and Rehabilitation. 2018;**99**(12):2621-2636

[25] Li CI, Malone KE, Daling JR. Differences in breast cancer stage, treatment, and survival by race and ethnicity. Archives of Internal Medicine. 2003;**163**(1):49-56

[26] Loh SY, Musa AN. Methods to improve rehabilitation of patients following breast cancer surgery: a review of systematic reviews. Breast Cancer: Targets and Therapy. 2015;7:81

[27] Guinan EM, Connolly EM, Hussey J. Exercise training in breast cancer survivors: a review of trials examining anthropometric and obesity-related biomarkers of breast cancer risk. Physical Therapy Reviews. 2013;**18**(2):79-89

[28] Ahles TA, Saykin AJ, Furstenberg CT, Cole B, Mott LA, Skalla K, et al. Neuropsychologic impact of standard-dose systemic chemotherapy in long-term survivors of breast cancer and lymphoma. Journal of Clinical Oncology. 2002;**20**(2):485-493

[29] Craddock RB, Adams PF, Usui WM, Mitchell L. An intervention to increase use and effectiveness of self-care measures for breast cancer chemotherapy patients. Cancer Nursing. 1999;**22**(4):312-319

[30] Naraphong W, Lane A, Schafer J, Whitmer K, Wilson BR. Exercise intervention for fatigue-related symptoms in Thai women with breast cancer: A pilot study. Nursing & Health Sciences. 2015;**17**:33-41

[31] Irwin ML, McTiernan JE, Manson CA, Thomson B, Sternfeld B, Stefanick ML, et al. Physical activity and survival in postmenopausal women with breast cancer: results from the women's health initiative. Cancer Prevention Research (Philadelphia, Pa.). 2011;**4**(4):522-529

[32] Pastakia K, Kumar S. Exercise parameters in the management of breast cancer: a systematic review of randomized controlled trials.

Physiotherapy Research International. 2011;**16**(4):237-244

[33] McNeely ML, Courneya KS. Exercise programs for cancer-related fatigue: evidence and clinical guidelines. Journal of the National Comprehensive Cancer Network. 2010;**8**(8):945-953